P9-EDW-146

Research in Athletic Training

POINT LOMA NAZARENE UNIVERSITY
RYAN LIBRARY
3900 LOMALAND DRIVE
SAN DIEGO, CALIFORNIA 92106-2899

613.71
I47r
03/03

Research in Athletic Training

Christopher D. Ingersoll, PhD, ATC, FACSM
Professor and Chair, Athletic Training Department
Indiana State University
Terre Haute, Indiana

POINT LOMA NAZARENE UNIVERSITY
WITHDRAWN
RYAN LIBRARY

SLACK

INCORPORATED

An innovative information, education and management company
6900 Grove Road • Thorofare, NJ 08086

Publisher: John H. Bond
Editorial Director: Amy E. Drummond
Assistant Editor: April C. Johnson

Copyright © 2001 by SLACK Incorporated

All rights reserved. No part of this book may be reproduced, stored in a retrieval system or transmitted in any form or by any means, electronic, mechanical, photocopying, recording or otherwise, without written permission from the publisher, except for brief quotations embodied in critical articles and reviews.

The procedures and practices described in this book should be implemented in a manner consistent with the professional standards set for the circumstances that apply in each specific situation. Every effort has been made to confirm the accuracy of the information presented and to correctly relate generally accepted practices. The author, editor, and publisher cannot accept responsibility for errors or exclusions or for the outcome of the application of the material presented herein. There is no expressed or implied warranty of this book or information imparted by it.

The work SLACK publishes is peer reviewed. Prior to publication, recognized leaders in the field, educators, and clinicians provide important feedback on the concepts and content that we publish. We welcome feedback on this work.

Printed in the United States of America.

Library of Congress Cataloging-in-Publication Data

Ingersoll, Christopher D
    Research in athletic training/Christopher Ingersoll.
       p. cm.
    Includes bibliographical references and index.
    ISBN 1-55642-439-6 (alk. paper)
     1. Physical education and training--Research. I. Title.

GV361 .I652 2001
796--dc21

                                        Library of Congress Control Number: 2001031371

Published by: SLACK Incorporated
                 6900 Grove Road
                 Thorofare, NJ 08086 USA
                 Telephone: 856-848-1000
                 Fax: 856-853-5991
                 www.slackbooks.com

Contact SLACK Incorporated for more information about other books in this field or about the availability of our books from distributors outside the United States.

Authorization to photocopy items for internal or personal use, or the internal or personal use of specific clients, is granted by SLACK Incorporated, provided that the appropriate fee is paid directly to Copyright Clearance Center, 222 Rosewood Drive, Danvers, MA 01923 USA, 978-750-8400. Prior to photocopying items for educational classroom use, please contact the CCC at the address above. Please reference Account Number 9106324 for SLACK Incorporated's Professional Book Division.
For further information on CCC, check CCC Online at the following address: http://www.copyright.com.

Last digit is print number: 10   9   8   7   6   5   4   3   2   1

CONTENTS

ACKNOWLEDGMENTS

Antoine de Saint-Exupéry said, "If you want to build a ship, don't drum up people together to collect wood and don't assign them tasks and work, but rather teach them to long for the endless immensity of the sea." Ken Knight instilled my love for the "sea." Now that I'm adrift I have one question, "What do I do now?" Seriously though, I am very grateful for having met Ken. He was the first person who really encouraged me to ask "Why?" Chapters Four and Eight are largely based on works we developed together.

I would like to acknowledge my colleagues at Indiana State University, Terre Haute, through the years; they have all impacted my thinking about research: Robert S. Behnke, HSD, ATC (Ret.); Mitchell L. Cordova, PhD, ATC; Mark Merrick, PhD, ATC; Kenneth L. Knight, PhD, ATC; John Kovaleski, PhD, ATC; Catherine L. Stemmans, PhD, ATC; Michelle A. Sandrey, PhD, ATC; David Ralston, MS, ATC; Lori Vancza, MS, ATC; Troy Hershman, MS, ATC; and Michelle Freeman, MS, ATC. Also, I would like to thank Brent Mangus, EdD, ATC, my colleague at the University of Nevada, Las Vegas, who helped shape me in the early part of my academic career.

Likewise, I have had the great privilege to work with the top scholars in our field while serving on the Research Committee and Board of Directors of the National Athletic Trainers' Association (NATA) Foundation, the Post-Certification Graduate Education Committee, and Executive Committee of the NATA Education Council. My interaction with these folks has greatly influenced the way I think about research in athletic training.

I must express my gratitude to my students over the years in ATTR 691: Research Methods in Athletic Training. Thanks for letting me try this stuff out on you.

This project could not have been completed without the help of graduate assistants who helped me collect information and/or read and reviewed numerous drafts of the manuscript: J. Ty Hopkins, PhD, ATC; B. Andrew Krause, MS, ATC; Riann Palmieri, MS, ATC; Marcus Stone, MS, ATC; Nikki Livecchi, MS, ATC; Jeff Otte, MS, ATC; and Kristin Kaufmann, ATC.

Marje Albohm, MS, ATC, recruited me to write this volume of the *Athletic Training Library*. I have never learned how to say "no" to Marje, who is the most dynamic leader you will ever meet. Amy Drummond and Kate Buczko from SLACK Incorporated were very patient with my "anal retentiveness" and "schizophrenia" during this project. Thanks Amy and Kate.

I extend my deepest love and appreciation to my family. Their daily sacrifices allow me to pursue my passion. Thanks Mary, Kayla, TJ, and Tommy.

ABOUT THE AUTHOR

Christopher D. Ingersoll's interest in athletic training research began during his undergraduate studies at Marietta College, Marietta, Ohio. His interest blossomed while a masters student at Indiana State University. He later earned a PhD in Biomechanics with a minor in Research and Statistics at the University of Toledo, Ohio.

In his first academic position at the University of Nevada, Las Vegas, he was involved in developing the Sports Injury Research Center. He then moved on to Indiana State University and assumed the role of director of the undergraduate athletic training education program. During his career at Indiana State, he has served as graduate program director, director of the Sports Injury Research Laboratory, chair of the Athletic Training Department, and is currently Interim Dean of the School of Graduate Studies. He has authored or coauthored over 100 peer-reviewed publications and nearly 150 international and national professional presentations. He has also served on nearly 100 thesis and dissertations committees.

Dr. Ingersoll has served the National Athletic Trainers' Association (NATA) Research and Education Foundation as a member; vice chair and chair of the Research Committee; vice president of the foundation; and currently as Foundation President and Chair of the Executive Committee. He was inaugural chair and is currently a member of the NATA Education Council Post-Certification Graduate Education Committee. He serves as editor for the *Journal of Sport Rehabilitation*. Further, he has served as an associate editor and is currently on the editorial board of the *Journal of Athletic Training*. He also serves on editorial boards for numerous other professional journals.

In his spare time, he enjoys racquetball, golf, and playing with Dixie and Rocket (his boxers). Most of all, he enjoys being with his wife, Mary, and children, Kayla, TJ, and Tommy. He doesn't like to eat tomatoes (and he has a good reason why).

FOREWORD

Athletic training research activity has increased dramatically in recent years and is becoming increasingly recognized as an important topic in athletic training education. Despite this increase, few materials are available that emphasize the specific needs of the athletic training student contemplating research. Christopher Ingersoll takes a strong step toward filling this void with the text, *Research in Athletic Training*. As the title indicates, Dr. Ingersoll focuses on issues specifically related to the profession of athletic training. This approach addresses the need for a unique research base, developed from within the profession, to link athletic trainers' skills to underlying theory.

The author is very well known and respected within the profession, and this text will be well received in accredited athletic training programs. *Research in Athletic Training* is not only a guide to developing the research project but also presents a philosophy of research for the athletic training student. Chapters One, Three, and Four challenge the student to contemplate why research is done, what is one's responsibility when conducting research, and what it means to be scholarly; all central notions underlying the research process. Chapters Two and Five through Nine take the reader through the fundamentals of conceptualizing, organizing, analyzing, producing, publishing, and fiscally supporting the research product, while Chapter Ten focuses on the place of research in the athletic training curriculum. The text is replete with examples familiar to the athletic training student.

This book will find favor in many accredited undergraduate and graduate athletic training programs, especially in programs where students are initially exposed to research.

Research in Athletic Training addresses a profession with a growing emphasis on the importance of systematic analysis; hence, Dr. Ingersoll's work can go a long way toward promoting a research culture in athletic training education.

Louis R. Osternig, PhD, ATC
University of Oregon
College of Arts and Sciences
Department of Exercise and Movement Science
Eugene, Oregon

PREFACE

I wrote this text for athletic trainers and athletic training students. I suspect that not all parts will be equally important to all athletic trainers or athletic training students. My hope is that this text might catalyze, in some small way, our movement to foster a research culture in athletic training.

The text grew from my Research in Athletic Training class notes over the years. I found that I needed to supplement the information provided in the textbook I used. The supplements were items that either expanded areas that were relevant to athletic training but were not covered well in available texts or items that helped present research in a context that made sense to athletic training students. My experience has been that copious use of examples was helpful in the classroom, so I tried to include some in the text.

Because of its origins, this text should work well as a supplement for undergraduate or graduate research classes. I also wrote with the practicing scholar and scholarly practitioner in mind. I hope that this volume serves as a cursory roadmap to research for these individuals. This text may also be used as a supplemental text in other classes, clinical courses, or seminars. Finally, it may be used as a compulsory reading assignment for students entering athletic training education programs; after all, they are the newest members of our research culture.

It was very important to me to present this information in a user-friendly format. Consequently, I chose to write in the first person (see Chapter Eight for more on why I did this). My hope is that this approach makes the material more inviting and personal. If this approach does not help, then I sincerely apologize.

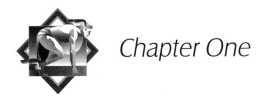

Chapter One

Why Do Research?

"Research is what I'm doing when I don't know what I'm doing." —*Wernher von Braun*

"Why do research?" is an important professional question. Most responsible practitioners and scholars will concur that research is important, but they may have some difficulty stating exactly why. To really buy into a research culture as a profession, we must be able to clearly and concisely answer this question and believe in what we say. Many relevant research texts[1-6] explain research and how to do it. I was unable to find any that explained why it is necessary or important to do research.

Perhaps the answer to this question is simply an assumption we all make. Perhaps it is diffusely presented in all of the scholarly work we do. Maybe it was covered in class the day I wasn't there. Regardless, I will make my attempt at directly answering this question and hope for continuing dialogue on the topic.

Conducting research is important for the following reasons:
- To develop new knowledge
- To improve our problem-solving skills
- To enhance our standing as professionals
- To improve the standard of care we provide
- To promote faster change and progress in the profession
- To develop our own body of knowledge
- To be viewed as experts in the health care of physically active people

DEVELOPING NEW KNOWLEDGE

New knowledge can be developed through trial and error. Without being subjected to the rigors of the scientific method, solutions derived from trial and error are more prone to inaccuracies. Research involves a systematic way of evaluating problems and introduces a comprehensive peer-review system. In short, knowledge developed using the scientific method is likely, but not guaranteed, to be more accurate than knowledge derived from other methods.

Ideas for new knowledge can come from anywhere. While the systematic process of the scientific method protects the accuracy of results as much as humanly possible, it does not directly encourage creativity in thinking. Ideally, development of new knowledge comes from creative and responsible practitioners and scholars through whatever method suits them. Determining whether these ideas are true or appropriate is best left to the rigors of the scientific method through research.

IMPROVING PROBLEM-SOLVING SKILLS

Learning about and practicing research not only allows us to develop our knowledge base, but they also make us better decision-makers. This is the single most noticeable trait I observe in graduate students as they proceed through their programs. While most do not come out of their master's degree program wishing to pursue a career in research, they are much more effective critical thinkers. They are much more likely to question existing methods, requiring others to provide support for the methods they use, and seek out support for their own methods. As such, they are more insistent on using methods that are supported by research. The better students even become critical of recommendations made in the literature based on inaccuracies in research design, statistical analysis, or even generalizations. In short, they become more iconoclastic in a professionally healthy way (an iconoclast is one who attacks traditional ideas or institutions).

IMPROVING PROFESSIONAL STANDING

Our professional standing is enhanced through research. Other health care professionals will judge us on the content of our educational curricula and how we are contributing to our own knowledge base without ever seeing what we actually do (I am going to focus on the research part of this issue). Professionals pay attention to where research is coming from and the quality of the research, as well as the author's credentials. When high-quality research is performed by athletic trainers, certified (ATCs), others notice.

The academic community will also evaluate us on our scholarly contributions to the profession. Athletic training education programs are housed in colleges and universities. Respect in the academy comes the same way for all professions—scholarly contributions. If we wish to continue to house our academic programs in institutions of higher learning, we need to play by their rules. This includes being responsible stewards for our knowledge base, promoting scholarship, and being scholarly (see Chapter Four for more on scholarship).

IMPROVING THE STANDARD OF CARE

The standard of care we provide will improve through research. Systematically asking and answering questions allows us to continually improve our understanding of what we do. The more we understand the effects of our interventions, the more effective they become. Physically active people get better faster and more completely now than they did 20 years ago because of research. Patients expect practitioners to continually search for better methods of treatment; therefore, we are obligated to do so.

PROMOTING CHANGE AND PROGRESS

Change and progress will come faster with ongoing improvements in our knowledge base. Numerous professional advancements in athletic training have come from our involvement in research. Consider the way we rehabilitate anterior cruciate ligament (ACL) reconstruction patients, evaluate sensorimotor deficits, or rationalize using cold for acute injuries. Without research, the progress seen in these areas would not occur. Worse yet, substandard, untested, and potentially hazardous methods could be used instead of more appropriate ones. Without research, change could certainly come but not necessarily progress.

DEVELOPING OUR BODY OF KNOWLEDGE

We must take responsibility for developing our own body of knowledge. If we do not, someone else will do it for us. Allowing this to happen presents two major problems:

- If others can do our research, why can't they perform our duties?
- Others will direct how we practice (ie, we will become technicians and lose our status as professionals).

Everyone must assume responsibility for developing our body of knowledge (see Chapter Three for more on responsibility for building our knowledge base).

EXPERTISE

If we are doing cutting-edge research, we become the experts in the health care of physically active people. The public, media, and health care profession identify experts by the quality of care provided. Quality of care provided is determined by the quality of the research performed to develop it. Being identified as experts improves employment opportunities, compensation, and funding opportunities for continued research.

In summary, the advantages of living in a research culture afford the following benefits:

- Having our own clearly identified body of knowledge
- Improving health care for the physically active
- Being unquestionably identified as professionals, not technicians
- Enhancing respect among the medical and allied health professions
- Receiving better pay
- Receiving better employment opportunities
- Receiving third-party reimbursement

REFERENCES

1. Ackerman WB, Lohnes PR. *Research Methods for Nurses.* New York: McGraw-Hill; 1981.
2. Bailey DM. *Research for the Health Professional: A Practical Guide.* 2nd ed. Philadelphia, Pa: FA Davis; 1997.
3. Neutens JJ, Rubinson L. *Research Techniques for the Health Sciences.* 2nd ed. Boston, Mass: Allyn and Bacon; 1997.
4. Shelley SI. *Research Methods in Nursing and Health.* Boston, Mass: Little, Brown and Co; 1984.
5. Thomas JR, Nelson JK. *Research Methods in Physical Activity.* 3rd ed. Champaign, Ill: Human Kinetics; 1996.
6. Wiersma W. *Research Methods in Education: An Introduction.* 6th ed. Boston, Mass: Allyn and Bacon; 1995.

Chapter Two

Research Areas
in Athletic Training

"Since our profession is still young, there are many unanswered questions regarding our clinical techniques and the validity of our instructional methods." —Louis R. Osternig

Athletic trainers should publish and present information that is important to the profession. Identification of research areas is important for ensuring that the whole spectrum of athletic training is being advanced. We have described educational competencies[1] for athletic training and the domains of athletic training practice.[2] Educational competencies represent what we feel is important to teach student athletic trainers. The practice domains represent the specific tasks that athletic trainers perform in their practices. In either situation, we have identified areas of our profession that we feel are important and, as a result, have identified areas that we think deserve study. We have also identified a knowledge base in which we have a professional responsibility to develop.

TYPES OF ATHLETIC TRAINING RESEARCH

Although numerous publications contain athletic training-related research, the *Journal of Athletic Training* is the largest and most representative. The *Journal of Athletic Training* publishes the following types of articles: original research, literature reviews, case reports, clinical techniques, and communications. These articles represent the way we present our research. Not all athletic training literature is presented in the *Journal of Athletic Training*, but it should be representative of what athletic trainers are studying and, hence, what we think is important.

BREAKDOWN OF RESEARCH TYPES

Tables 2-1 and 2-2 present breakdowns of article types by educational competencies and practice domains, respectively, in the *Journal of Athletic Training* during the period from 1992 to 1998. I included teaching/pedagogy to both educational competencies and practice domains. How we teach our students is an important area of inquiry. These tables are snapshots of what we have chosen to study in the recent past. Reviewing this data can roughly identify areas in which we have committed great effort and areas that we have not adequately addressed.

Slightly more than half (53%) of the articles published were original research articles, which means that half of what we publish is new knowledge and half is synthesis of existing knowledge. This seems like a good ratio that we ought to preserve or even tip toward the new knowledge side.

Table 2-1

Breakdown of Journal of Athletic Training (1992-1998) Article Types by Educational Competencies (N, % Total)

Educational Domain	Article Type					
	Original Research	Literature Review	Case Reports	Clinical Techniques	Communications	Total
Risk Management and Injury Prevention	38, 11.62%	3, 0.92%	0, 0.00%	11, 3.36%	2, 0.61%	54, 16.51%
Pathology of Injuries and Illnesses	9, 2.75%	4, 1.22%	0, 0.00%	0, 0.00%	0, 0.00%	13, 3.98%
Assessment and Evaluation	13, 3.98%	9, 2.75%	31, 9.48%	7, 2.14%	1, 0.31%	61, 18.65%
Acute Care of Injuries and Illnesses	4, 1.22%	2, 0.61%	1, 0.31%	10, 3.06%	1, 0.31%	18, 5.50%
Pharmacology	3, 0.92%	5, 1.53%	1, 0.31%	0, 0.00%	2, 0.61%	11, 3.36%
Therapeutic Modalities	38, 11.62%	0, 0.00%	1, 0.31%	1, 0.31%	0, 0.00%	40, 12.23%
Therapeutic Exercise	26, 7.95%	0, 0.00%	6, 1.83%	11, 3.36%	0, 0.00%	43, 13.15%
General Medical Conditions and Disabilities	2, 0.61%	6, 1.83%	1, 0.31%	1, 0.31%	0, 0.00%	10, 3.06%
Nutritional Aspects of Injury and Illness	1, 0.31%	3, 0.92%	0, 0.00%	0, 0.00%	1, 0.31%	5, 1.53%
Psychosocial Intervention and Referral	8, 2.45%	1, 0.31%	0, 0.00%	2, 0.61%	3, 0.92%	14, 4.28%
Health Care Administration	19, 5.81%	3, 0.92%	0, 0.00%	3, 0.92%	7, 2.14%	32, 9.79%
Professional Development and Responsibilities	1, 0.31%	3, 0.92%	0, 0.00%	1, 0.31%	4, 1.22%	9, 2.75%
Teaching/Pedagogy	13, 3.98%	1, 0.31%	0, 0.00%	1, 0.31%	2, 0.61%	17, 5.20%
Total	175, 53.52%	40, 12.23%	41, 12.54%	48, 14.68%	23, 7.03%	327, 100.00%

Table 2-2

BREAKDOWN OF JOURNAL OF ATHLETIC TRAINING (1992-1998) ARTICLE TYPES BY PRACTICE DOMAINS (N, %TOTAL)

Practice Domain	Article Type					
	Original Research	Literature Review	Case Reports	Clinical Techniques	Communi-cations	Total
Prevention	45, 13.76%	6, 1.83%	0, 0.00%	11, 3.36%	2, 0.61%	64, 19.57%
Recognition, Evaluation, and Assessment	21, 6.42%	20, 6.12%	32, 9.79%	8, 2.45%	1, 0.31%	82, 25.08%
Immediate Care	3, 0.92%	2, 0.61%	1, 0.31%	8, 2.45%	1, 0.31%	15, 4.59%
Treatment, Rehabilitation, and Reconditioning	68, 20.80%	5, 1.53%	8, 2.45%	15, 4.59%	3, 0.92%	99, 30.28%
Organization and Administration	21, 6.42%	3, 0.92%	0, 0.00%	4, 1.22%	10, 3.06%	38, 11.62%
Professional Development and Responsibility	3, 0.92%	3, 0.92%	0, 0.00%	1, 0.31%	4, 1.22%	11, 3.36%
Teaching/Pedagogy	14, 4.28%	1, 0.31%	0, 0.00%	1, 0.31%	2, 0.61%	18, 5.50%
Total	175, 53.52%	40, 12.23%	41, 12.54%	48, 14.68%	23, 7.03%	327, 100.00%

Table 2-3

PERCENTAGE OF PAPERS IN JOURNAL OF ATHLETIC TRAINING AND PERCENTAGE OF TIME SPENT ON PRACTICE DOMAINS

Domain	% *JAT* articles	% practice time[2]
Prevention	19.57	15.44
Recognition, Evaluation, and Prevention	25.08	22.87
Immediate Care	4.59	17.98
Treatment, Rehabilitation, and Reconditioning	30.28	25.61
Organization and Administration	11.62	10.75
Professional Development and Responsibility	3.36	7.60

THERAPEUTIC MODALITIES AND THERAPEUTIC EXERCISE

More than one-third of original research papers were in the therapeutic modalities and therapeutic exercise educational competencies or in the treatment, rehabilitation, and reconditioning practice domain; they represent a full 20% of all articles published. Accordingly, we spend about 25% of our time in this area (Table 2-3). Certainly, the amount of time spent on rehabilitation varies from setting to setting. Inquiry into these areas should continue, but we need to develop scholars that will contribute to other areas as well.

RISK MANAGEMENT AND INJURY PREVENTION

The risk management and injury prevention educational competency and the prevention practice domain were the second most frequently published areas. Many of these papers involved the effects of taping and bracing techniques; articles evaluating injury prevention programming were absent. Athletic trainers take great pride in their role in injury prevention, but we have done little to study our effectiveness in this area. Scholars in this area of inquiry are greatly needed. Many young professionals have asked what area of study they should pursue in their doctoral work. My suggestion: "First and foremost, do what interests you, but a good dose of epidemiology wouldn't hurt." Epidemiology provides the tools that begin to answer questions in the areas of risk management and injury prevention.

Knowledge in the area of risk management and injury prevention may also be important to support, or even pay for, our services. If we want someone to pay us to provide risk management or injury prevention services, we will need to show them that our methods work.

IMMEDIATE CARE

There is a large disparity in the percentage of time spent on immediate care and the percentage of articles published in that area. Clearly, we share a lot of information in this area with other professionals, but we need to step up our research efforts in this area to match its importance in our jobs.

Studies of the safety and effectiveness of emergency care procedures we employ will be essential in demonstrating that they work. Further, if we are to continue improving and refining our level of care in this area, we need to propose new approaches and make sure they result in improved service.

NEW EDUCATIONAL COMPETENCIES

New areas represented in the educational competencies (pathology of injuries and illnesses, acute care of injuries and illnesses, pharmacology, general medical conditions and disabilities, nutritional aspects of injury and illness, and psychosocial intervention and referral) are poorly represented in our literature. If we continue identifying these as important educational competencies, we need to do a much better job of studying them. Identifying topics as integral to our profession without contributing to the knowledge base in that area is professionally irresponsible. Scholars are also needed in these areas but are understandably not yet developed.

CASE REPORTS

Well-done case reports are essential. There were 41 case reports in the *Journal of Athletic Training* during the 7-year period examined, which comes out to an average of less than six unique cases published per year. I would suggest that there are more than six unique cases per year worthy of sharing with athletic trainers (I do understand that case reports may be presented in journals other than the *Journal of Athletic Training*). There were averages of 24 case reports presented each of the past 3 years at the annual NATA meeting. These cases were presented to a relatively small audience; hence, the potential impact of sharing the unique information contained in these case reports is greatly minimized. We need to share our unique cases with each other more often as journal articles, not just as presentations.

CLINICAL TECHNIQUE REPORTS

I make the same plea for more clinical technique reports. Clinical techniques supported by literature and logic should be presented more frequently. Again, if we do not share our ideas, their impact is minimized. If you have a highly effective clinical technique that you never share, relatively few patients will benefit. If you use your technique on your patients for your entire career, you help hundreds of people. If you share it in a publication, thousands or hundreds of thousands may benefit. Failure to share such valuable information may be considered a breach of responsibility on the part of a professional person.

SUGGESTED NOMENCLATURE FOR
RESEARCH AREAS IN ATHLETIC TRAINING

Athletic training research presented in publications is often categorized by the educational competency or practice domain it covers (as I have done above and as done by the *Journal of Athletic Training* and other reputable journals), or by the research design used and the intent of the study (as done by many funding agencies, including the NATA Foundation). Currently, the NATA Foundation categorizes research as follows:

- *Basic Science*—includes controlled laboratory studies in the subdisciplines of exercise physiology, biomechanics, and motor behavior, among others, that relate to athletic training and sports medicine.
- *Clinical Studies*—include assessments of the validity, reliability, and efficacy of clinical procedures, rehabilitation protocols, injury prevention programs, surgical techniques, and so on.
- *Educational Research*—a broad category ranging from basic surveys to detailed athletic training/sports medicine curriculum development. Studies in this category will generally include assessments of student learning, teaching effectiveness (didactic or clinical), educational materials, and curriculum development.
- *Sports Injury Epidemiology*—includes studies of injury patterns among athletes. These studies generally encompass large-scale data collection and analysis. Surveys and questionnaires may be classified in this category but are more likely to come under the Observation/Informational Studies category.
- *Observation/Informational Studies*—include studies involving surveys, questionnaires, and descriptive programs, among others, that relate to athletic training and sports medicine.

These definitions have essentially served us well in the past; however, I believe that inadequate emphasis is placed on clinical research. Most scholars would not share our definition of basic science. Nearly all of the studies submitted under this area have clinical intent if not direct clinical applicability. Likewise, these definitions represent a mix of categories represented by the type of design used, and others represent a general intent of the study. I suggest that we begin to evolve into a system of identifying the types of research in athletic training based on the type of design used. Consider the following categories, adapted from the *International Review Board Guidebook*[3]:

- *Observation*—behavioral research consisting of observing people in public places.
- *Record Reviews and Historical Studies*—studies involving the use of public or private records. Such studies use existing records to document the past.
- *Surveys, Questionnaires, and Interviews*—research using a systematically developed tool (survey, questionnaire, or interview) to collect descriptive information from or draw inferences about a sample or population.
- *Epidemiological Studies*—studies attempting to identify risk factors for particular diseases, conditions, or behaviors, or risks that result from particular causes, such as environmental or industrial agents.
- *Case-Control Studies*—studies in which persons with a specific condition (the cases) and persons without the condition (the controls) are selected to participate. The proportions of cases and controls with certain characteristics are then compared. For example, the number of female athletes who have suffered ACL tears and have small intercondylar notches is compared to the number of female athletes who have not suffered ACL injuries with small intercondylar notches.
- *Prospective Studies*—studies designed to observe events (eg, diseases, behavioral or physiological responses) that may occur after the subjects have been identified. All concurrently controlled clinical trials are prospective.

- *Clinical Trials*—research designed to assess the safety and efficacy of new drugs, devices, treatments, or preventive measures in humans by comparing two or more interventions or regimens.

The model discussed here did not include educational research—a category we may wish to add. The focus of this model is to present ways to study the practice of our profession, not so much the teaching of it. The study of how we teach our students is very important and should, of course, continue.

Great emphasis is placed on designs that use injured or ill subjects. Although research on normal subjects is not excluded, emphasis should be placed on studying injured or ill subjects. That is how we will ultimately begin to understand the effectiveness of our interventions.

We must clearly define our research areas because they represent what we view as our body of knowledge. If we cannot clearly define them, we do not have a clear body of knowledge. If we do not have a clear body of knowledge, we do not have a clearly identified profession. If we do not have a clearly identified profession, we cannot call ourselves professionals. The ability to call ourselves professionals is essential. We must expend much thought into this question in order to effectively evolve athletic training.

REFERENCES

1. National Athletic Trainers' Association. *Athletic Training Educational Competencies.* 3rd ed. Dallas, Tex: National Athletic Trainers' Association; 1999.

2. National Athletic Trainers' Association Board of Certification. *Role Delineation Study.* 4th ed. Omaha, Neb: National Athletic Trainers' Association Board of Certification; 1999.

3. *The Institutional Review Board Guidebook (IRB Guidebook—revised 1993).* Available at: http://ohrp.osophs.dhhs.gov/irb/irb_guidebook.htm. Accessed July 18, 2000.

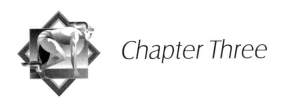

Chapter Three

Responsibility for Building the Athletic Training Knowledge Base

"We live on an island surrounded by a sea of ignorance. As our island of knowledge grows, so does the shore of our ignorance." —John A. Wheeler

All athletic trainers are responsible for building the knowledge base in athletic training, but most are not doing their part. Some possible reasons for this include lack of knowledge, job site barriers, and attitudinal barriers.[1]

LACK OF KNOWLEDGE

Lack of knowledge can be overcome. Research is like a game: in order to win, you need to know the rules. Like with any complex game, very few people are completely knowledgeable about all of the rules. Comprehension of the basics is enough to get started. Knowledge increases with experience. The courage to get started is a great barrier.

Some specific issues related to lack of knowledge include[1]:
- Unfamiliarity with the research process
- Unfamiliarity with the use of statistics
- Lack of research ideas
- Unwillingness to make research a higher priority
- Lack of outside funding
- Stringent publication requirements
- Lack of research consultants

Unfamiliarity with the Research Process

Unfamiliarity with the research process is an educational problem (see Chapter Ten for suggestions on teaching the research process). The research process must be introduced to students during their undergraduate experience. If it is not presented in a student's undergraduate program, it must be featured in graduate experiences. If our educational experiences are presented properly, this can become a nonissue.

For those athletic trainers who have completed their formal education, I suggest starting with Chapter Five in this text and continuing to read research texts. Reading about research, learning its language, and embracing its value to our profession helps ease it into our everyday professional lives. Do not be afraid to consult those involved in research to enhance your own knowledge.

Programming at state, district, and national meetings could also address research issues. Symposia and workshops could be presented to athletic trainers of all levels of involvement in research. Our professional organizations ought to pay more attention to these topic areas.

Unfamiliarity with the Use of Statistics

This problem could be resolved in the same way as unfamiliarity with the research process. Statistics bring out the math phobia in everyone. If you can add, subtract, multiply, divide, and use exponentiation (a number to the power of some other number; eg, 2^3), then the necessary math skills for understanding statistics are accessible to you. The difficult part of statistics is logic, not math. Understanding when to use statistical analyses requires logical thinking.

You may wish to use a statistical consultant to help you with your research. If you do, consult one early in the process, not at the end. A statistician cannot fix faulty design with a particular statistical analysis. I contend that more serious problems occur as a result of faulty research designs than use of inappropriate statistical analyses.

An important point to remember is that you will most likely not have to compute statistical analyses by hand. Statistics software is readily available. A computer will do the calculations. Your job is to interpret their meaning. This is not always easy, but it is doable.

Lack of Research Ideas

I doubt that good athletic trainers do not have research ideas. Rather, they may not be trained to recognize them when presented. If you allow yourself to ask some of the following questions, you cannot help but encounter unanswered questions. Unanswered questions are the basis of research ideas. Ask the following questions regularly:
- Which method is better?
- Why did(n't) that treatment work?
- How did that treatment work?
- Is there a better way?
- How did this injury occur?
- Why am I doing it this way?

Athletic trainers have plenty of research ideas. The trick is to mine and refine them.

Unwillingness to Make Research a Higher Priority

This issue is listed under the heading Lack of Knowledge because I believe that lack of knowledge is the cause of this problem. Unwillingness to make research a higher priority means settling for the inferior methods of treatment that are currently available. Having the tools to improve patient care is invaluable. If the literature does not provide the answers to our questions, we have two choices: 1) wait until the thought passes and forget about improving patient care, or 2) try to answer the question ourselves. The latter is more difficult but more rewarding.

Lack of Outside Funding

Lack of outside funding is usually due to lack of knowledge to find and request funds. To get started in finding and requesting outside funding, refer to Chapter Nine in this text.

Stringent Publication Requirements

Fear of the stringent requirements for publishing research stems from unfamiliarity with the publication process. Communicating your ideas in professional journals is more like the language we use in our everyday practices than the jargon-laden, impossibly complex scientific journal article of myth. Refer to Chapter Eight for a jump-start in preparing journal articles. Many articles are returned to authors for corrections. This should not be viewed as punishment but rather a chance to fine-tune your article. A better article makes you look better. This is a win-win situation.

Sometimes articles are rejected. It happens to the best of us. Often, you can find a journal that is interested in your paper even though it was rejected elsewhere. If not, learn something from the experience. Look for the lesson in the experience after the initial anger has worn off! I have not met an experienced author yet who has not had a manuscript rejected at some point.

Lack of Research Consultants

The inability to locate a research consultant is a legitimate concern because some types of research require specialized knowledge. Locating a research consultant can be problematic. Development of an athletic training research network could help match interested parties with research consultants (see Building an Athletic Training Research Network in Chapter Six).

JOB SITE BARRIERS

All job sites present barriers to performing research. Even athletic trainers in institutions of higher learning encounter obstacles to research involvement. Some of these barriers include[1]:
- Lack of administrative financial support
- Lack of equipment and facilities
- Lack of administrative philosophical support
- Lack of library facilities
- Lack of consistent patient load
- Inability to give up revenue-producing time

These barriers can be overcome in many instances.

Lack of Administrative Financial Support

In general, I believe that research costs money. On the other hand, I also believe that money should not be a barrier to gaining desired knowledge. Often, research can be seamlessly worked into your daily work schedule. If your research involves collecting information from situations you encounter every day, then additional funds may not be necessary.

If your institution will not provide funds for your research, you may need to write a grant. See Chapter Nine in this text for a primer on writing a grant.

Lack of Equipment and Facilities

Expensive equipment and facilities are not always necessary for good research. In certain instances, specific pieces of equipment are needed to collect data. If the equipment is unavailable, it presents a barrier. Collaborating with the colleges/universities or medical facilities possessing the necessary equipment may help resolve these types of issues. Depending on the cost of the equipment, you may be able to secure it by writing a grant (see Chapter Nine).

Lack of Administrative Philosophical Support

Preventing professionals from performing their duty to advance the profession is exploitation. Institutions may or may not realize they are exploiting their employees. Often, athletic trainers are not viewed as professionals. When this occurs, administrators do not appreciate the need for professional responsibility to advance knowledge. Communicating with administrators is important in this regard. Discussing the direct and indirect advantages of developing the athletic training knowledge base is important. Educating administrators about athletic training will help them understand and appreciate the profession.

Lack of Library Facilities

This barrier becomes less of a problem as the Internet grows. Literature searches can be done for free (http://www.ncbi.nlm.nih.gov/PubMed/), and some articles can even be ordered through search engines (eg, www.Northernlight.com). I cannot remember the last time I was in the library except to pick up a book that I knew was in the library because I located it on the Internet.

Lack of Consistent Patient Load

Research can be hampered if you are studying a specific condition but do not examine a consistent flow of patients with that condition. A possible solution to this problem is to collaborate with others or develop a multisite research project. A research network for athletic trainers would be helpful in developing these efforts. Likewise, the study may need to stretch over several years to get the necessary number of subjects. Good answers are worth waiting for.

Inability to Give Up Revenue-Producing Time

Write a grant to buy the time spent on research. The institution is compensated for your time, and you can do the research. That is what research funds are for.

ATTITUDINAL BARRIERS

Attitudinal barriers are the most disconcerting to me. The most common attitudinal barriers are an unwillingness to invest the time and a lack of interest. I understand that we are all busy and research may add additional time burdens; however, can we be satisfied providing the same level of care for the next 20 years? Simply put, we are health care providers, and we have a responsibility to provide the best care possible. Sometimes that means we must make sacrifices to find or develop the necessary care.

As for lack of interest, refer to the section entitled Lack of Knowledge in this chapter. The two are connected.

ROLE OF THE ATHLETIC TRAINER IN RESEARCH

Albright[2] identified the following research roles for an athletic trainer:
- Supervisor of injury data collection
- Source of performance and examination measurements
- Clinical coordinator in multicenter studies
- Clinical consultant to a research team
- Public relations liaison with parents and coaches
- Research team leader in selected studies in which a physician is not required for diagnosis and treatment responsibilities

I agree that all of these roles are important for athletic trainers to play. Involvement in physicians' research is of value to both physicians and athletic trainers; however, I believe that athletic trainers need to play the role of conceptualizer as often as possible. This should be the first role on our list. Physicians and other health care providers will benefit from the research we do.

Athletic training should have scholars with their own area of inquiry. This means they must complete the educational training necessary; have a comprehensive knowledge of their content area, research design, and statistics; and have a directed and sustainable line of research. In other words, we must be more than data collectors: we must be the developers and guardians of our body of knowledge. Not all athletic trainers will choose this career path. We need to have most of our professionals actively engaged in the practice of athletic training, but we must also have scholars who make it their primary business to do research. This is healthy for the profession.

Most importantly, by doing our own research we are taking responsibility for advancing our own profession. This is paramount if we want to be considered professionals. In order for us to be considered professionals, we all have to participate.

REFERENCES

1. Ballin AJ, Breslin WH, Wierenga KAS, Shepard KF. Research in physical therapy: philosophy, barriers to involvement, and use among California physical therapists. *Phys Ther.* 1980;60:888-895.
2. Albright JP. Role of the athletic trainer. *Am J Sports Med.* 1988;16(suppl1):S5-S9.

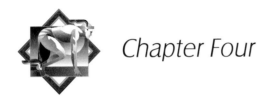

Chapter Four

Scholarship and Being Scholarly

"The test of a first-rate intelligence is the ability to hold two opposed ideas in the mind at the same time and still retain the ability to function." —F. Scott Fitzgerald

Scholarship is the process of advancing knowledge. Scholarship is attained by discovering new knowledge and original insights that add to the world's body of knowledge and understanding, integrating existing knowledge in one discipline with that of another discipline, and developing new and better means for describing, understanding, and presenting existing knowledge.[1] Scholarship delineates a profession from a trade.[2] The importance of scholarship in athletic training has been discussed several times during the past 15 years.[2-5]

Scholarship should be developed and carried out according to clearly articulated purposes and procedures consistent with disciplinary norms. It must contain some element of originality in the form of new knowledge, new understanding, fresh insight, or unique interpretation. Scholarly work must undergo critical review and acceptance by discerning peers for the purpose of verifying the nature and quality of its contribution.[6]

The most traditional and accepted way of satisfying the criteria is through publication in a recognized, peer reviewed, scholarly journal; however, acceptance for publication by a journal does not necessarily reflect quality.[1]

ELEMENTS OF SCHOLARSHIP

Scholarship is more than just research and writing. In order to fully understand the concept of scholarship, we need to understand knowledge, truth, and theory.

Knowledge

Knowledge consists of facts and theories that enable one to understand phenomena and to solve problems.[7] Knowledge can range from the simplest perception of an object to the most profound understanding of a complex theory.[1] Knowledge can be obtained from direct personal experience or from second-hand sources of information.[7] Knowledge is a personal interpretation of what might be the truth.

Truth

Truth is "the state of being; the case, fact; or the body of real things, events, and facts; actuality."[6] Truth should never be confused with opinion or belief, which portrays a person's attitude, because attitudes may or may not coincide with facts.[8] Truth is not relative. Beliefs, opinions, and theories may be relative but truth is not.

Theory

A theory is a generalization or series of generalizations by which we attempt to explain some phenomena in a systematic manner.[9] It is a deductively correct set of truths and beliefs. The criterion by which we judge a theory is not its truth or falsity, but rather its usefulness in stimulating thought and research. Theories sometimes decrease in usefulness in the light of new knowledge, and they are combined, replaced, and refined as more knowledge is made available. Theories are dynamic structures.[1]

Theories provide the framework for research. They:

- Serve as points of departure
- Help identify crucial factors
- Aid in defining the research problem
- Provide guides for systematizing and interrelating various facets of the research
- Identify gaps, weak points, and inconsistencies that indicate the need for additional research[1]

Theories can be used for synthesizing and explaining research results as follows:

- They allow one to combine ideas and individual bits of empirical information into a set of constructs that provide deeper understanding, broader meaning, and wider applicability.
- They attach meaning to facts and place them in proper perspective, thus providing needed information for revising or extending theory if necessary.
- They provide generalizations that can be tested and used in practical applications and further research.[1]

Data derive significance from the theory or theories into which they fit. Conversely, theories become acceptable to the extent that they enhance the meaning of the data through theory development. More adequate theories and unobstructed facts are secured; theory stimulates research, and conversely, research stimulates theory development and testing.[9] Confused theory based on partial or incomplete truth rather than the whole truth leads to techniques that are partially effective or ineffective.

ATTRIBUTES OF A SCHOLAR

Knight and Ingersoll[1] described scholarly attributes or characteristics as follows. A scholar:

1. Seeks to establish truth and develop new knowledge
   a. through original research
   b. by synthesizing and integrating established knowledge in a new or unique way
   c. by re-examining commonly held ideas, concepts, and theories to determine whether they are based on truth
2. Develops and refines theory
   a. bases one's research on theory and emphasizes what a set of data means in addition to how it looks, feels, appears, etc
   b. explains how one's research results relate to other known data and theories rather than leaving the results for others to interpret
3. Is focused on one's work
   a. has a specific area of investigation that narrows with time; a scholar's research interests do not randomly change from topic to topic
   b. is meticulous in detail
4. Is honest about one's work
   a. clearly admits assumptions upon which one's work is based, speculation about the meaning of the results, and the limitations of one's work and its applications
   b. understands that discovering truth is more important than convincing others that one's interpretations are correct

    c. is motivated by refining and expanding an area rather than protecting one's personal interpretation of the idea

    d. accepts truth as it becomes known, even if it contradicts one's previously held theories or ideas

5. Communicates ideas and stirs thinking

    a. is more interested in the quality of one's publications than the quantity of one's publications

    b. does not rush papers into publication but labors over them to improve their quality and readability

    c. knows that sounding "scholarly" is not as important as effectively communicating ideas; understands that using simple words often enhances reader and listener comprehension

    d. points out assumptions, limitations, and speculations in papers so that readers can clearly put the works into perspective

    e. is not afraid to stick one's neck out if data appear to conflict with accepted theory and ideas

    f. encourages others to join in searching for the truth

6. Is open-minded

    a. follows the philosophy of Francis Bacon: "Read not to contradict or refute, nor to accept and take for granted, but to weigh and consider."

    b. is willing to listen to alternatives with an open mind, is open enough that one can defend either the pro or con of an argument, and is willing to change positions as new truths are uncovered

    c. does not ignore data that do not fit expectations but rather seeks to integrate all truth

    d. recognizes the difference between true scholarship and pseudoscholarship

    e. knows that presenting information is not necessarily scholarship. For instance, most reliability studies testing the accuracy of instruments, product research, and technique articles are important pursuits; however, they are technical supports of scholarship, not scholarship itself. Scholars deepen and broaden theory.

TYPES OF SCHOLARS

Mosey[10] discussed scholarship in occupational therapy and divided scholars into two basic categories: scientists and philosophers. She described scientists as those who use research designs or theoretical information to accurately describe the physical world or to address specific practical problems and issues. She felt that scientists in occupational therapy focused their attention primarily on enhancing the scientific portion of the profession by:

- Formulating and refining the frames of reference used by the profession to guide evaluation and intervention relative to the multiple elements of human experience that constitute the profession's domain of concern
- Evaluating frames of reference relative to the safety, reliability, and validity of their guidelines for problem identification and the interpractitioner reliability of their guidelines for problem remediation; the safety, effectiveness, and efficiency of their use relative to various populations; when, how, and under what circumstances they are best used; and the optimal duration and frequency of their use
- Developing and refining screening tools, including establishing their reliability, validity, and, when appropriate, normative values
- Designing, conducting, and interpreting outcomes studies of occupational therapy programs involving the combined use of a variety of frames of reference in relation to persons with various diagnosed conditions

- Identifying and developing theoretical information needed by the profession either as an independent scientist or through directing the inquiry of scientists within whatever discipline is responsible for studying the phenomena of concern

Mosey[10] defined philosophers as persons who use the methods of scholarly inquiry and the various analytic techniques of philosophy to address the ideas, beliefs, values, assumptions, and arguments that are pivotal to a society's thinking, actions, and about which it has questions. Philosophers focus their attention on enhancing the profession's body of knowledge by:

- Identifying questions about, examining, clarifying, and, when deemed appropriate, making changes in statements regarding the profession's code of ethics, philosophical assumptions, and core values and attitudes
- Considering epistemological questions regarding the profession's body of knowledge, including what it is or should be and how it is or should be developed, organized, evaluated, and used
- Identifying, examining, clarifying, and taking positions on philosophical issues of concern to the profession for the ultimate purpose of enabling involved parties to make well-considered, wise decisions in resolving the issues

SCHOLARLY PRACTITIONERS

All professions need scholars. In clinical professions like athletic training most make their living practicing the profession rather than practicing in a laboratory. Clinicians can be scholarly, however. Consider the major attributes or characteristics of a scholar and how these attributes or characteristics can be expressed in a clinical setting.

Seeking Truth and Developing New Knowledge

Practitioners can perform original research (see Chapter Five), synthesize and integrate existing knowledge in new and unique ways, and re-examine commonly held ideas, concepts, and theories to determine whether they are based on truth. Clinician involvement in research is discussed in Chapter Five. The importance of athletic trainers contributing to our knowledge base cannot be overemphasized.

The best clinicians are always synthesizing and integrating existing knowledge in new and unique ways. Understanding existing knowledge comes from being an avid consumer of athletic training literature. Most of the literature in athletic training focuses on research using normal subjects. Injured athletes often respond differently to treatments than athletic training graduate students (the most commonly used subjects in athletic training research); therefore, clinicians must constantly attempt new ways to understand and implement the information learned. Sometimes things work differently in the clinic than in the laboratory. Do not be afraid to experiment.

Re-examining commonly held ideas, concepts, and theories should be done daily. Much of what we do clinically is based on strings of inductively derived premises. Often, one or more of the underlying premises of why we are doing something is incorrect. If a premise is found to be incorrect, often the conclusion needs to be changed. Because we cannot support everything we do clinically with research results, we must rely on reasoning; however, as we challenge our reasoning, we often discover ways to enhance our knowledge in that area. Uncovering false premises can lead to important areas of inquiry in the field.

As an example, I would like to discuss a premise I believe to be false about the effect of cryotherapy during rehabilitation. Improved functional state in an injured athlete following cold application, as with cryokinetics, has been attributed to alleviation of pain. The idea is that as pain is removed, muscle inhibition is removed. If muscle inhibition is removed, the patient can perform active exercise more effectively. We have learned in our laboratory, however, that muscle inhibition can occur in the absence of pain using a joint effusion model. We also know that the inhibition from this effusion can be removed with cryotherapy. Because there was no pain to begin with, removal of the pain could not have been the cause of disinhibition. Therefore, the premise that cold-induced hyperesthesia or analgesia is responsible for removing inhibition is not always true. If inhibition can be removed in the absence of pain, something else has to be partially responsible. Each time we undertake this type of questioning, we get closer to the truth of the matter.

Developing and Refining Theory

In order to develop and refine a theory, something must be known of an existing theory. Again, reading the literature helps. Clinicians can develop a theory by actually testing hypotheses in a study (see Chapter Five). Refinement of theory can be accomplished by implementing a current theory into practice. Most of the time, things do not work in the clinic the same way they work in the laboratory. Theory refinement can come from field-testing. Identification of clinical issues that effect implementation of ideas and theories is very important work.

Being Focused on One's Work

Being focused on a specific aspect of athletic training practice is not always possible for practitioners. Athletic trainers are, by nature, multiskilled clinicians. Therefore, knowledge must support all practice areas. Failure to focus on one aspect of practice is not a weakness for a practitioner, unless one is a specialist. As specialty areas develop in athletic training, we may see more people focusing on one area.

Being Honest about One's Work

Being honest about one's work extends beyond research. Being honest about why you select the clinical solutions you do is also important. Again, every clinician cannot be up-to-date on literature in every aspect of the profession. We sometimes do things because that is the way we were taught; this is OK. Being a scholarly clinician involves being honest about it. If you do something a certain way because that was how you were taught, say so. Clinicians cannot be expected to know everything or have a detailed rationale for everything they do. Scholarly clinicians are willing to admit this and seek information to remedy deficits in knowledge as needed.

Communicating Ideas and Stirring Thinking

Share your ideas with others. If they disagree with you, they are doing you and possibly themselves a favor. As others question our ideas, it presents opportunities to find weaknesses in our thinking. It is worse to leave an idea undiscussed and unrefined than to be wrong. When a flawed idea is exposed, the opportunity to rectify it is presented. Flawed ideas that are never discussed remain flawed. Patients do not benefit from flawed ideas. The most scholarly clinicians I know often start a sentence with, "I may be wrong, but I think…," and great discussions often follow.

Being Open-Minded

Things are not always as they seem. If we do not allow ourselves to see new or unique solutions, we can never find optimal methods of helping our patients. In sports medicine, it is sometimes difficult to be open-minded. Anything medical is susceptible to quackery. Anything related to sports is susceptible to great marketing with weak rationale (eg, the exercise equipment market). Sometimes the strangest approaches may be the best.

To amplify this point, I would like to share another personal experience. Return to our cryotherapy example earlier in the chapter in which pain removal may not be the mechanism for disinhibition.

We have found in our laboratory that cooling the axilla can facilitate the soleus muscle. While it does not facilitate the soleus as much as ankle cooling, it still causes substantial facilitation. If we wanted to incorporate functional activities in our rehabilitation, the patient may believe his or her ankle is too cold and stiff to do really vigorous exercise following cryotherapy. If we were able to disinhibit the musculature in the lower extremity by cooling the axilla, we could eliminate the feeling of stiffness in the ankle but still promote active exercise. Let us examine how a clinical recommendation could come out of this information: "Cool the armpit to remove muscle inhibition in the lower extremities." Most clinicians would view this recommendation with much criticism, as they should; however, there may be something to it. More work needs to be done before I would actually stand by this recommendation, but someday I may. If you hear me saying this, please be open-minded.

PROMOTING SCHOLARSHIP IN ATHLETIC TRAINING

The responsibility for promoting scholarship in athletic training is shared by many. The National Athletic Trainers' Association (NATA) has a responsibility to promote scholarship among its members. It does so by sponsoring a professional journal, the *Journal of Athletic Training*. The *Journal of Athletic Training* is the medium by which we can share our scholarship. It is our attempt to represent and share truth, knowledge, and theories within the field. The NATA has also provided funding over the years to support research studies. NATA has learned to solve problems using data and a scholarly approach. This attitude strengthens the athletic trainer's role in health care and enhances his or her status among other medical professionals. To learn more about the NATA and athletic training, visit their website at http://www.nata.org.

The NATA Research and Education Foundation also contributes to scholarship in the field. In fact, the foundation is, and should be, the major vehicle to support research and scholarship in the field of athletic training. The foundation provides a comprehensive research grants program to enhance research in and relevant to the profession. Free communication presentations at the NATA annual meeting and clinical symposia are sponsored by the foundation. Scholarships for undergraduate and graduate students are also provided by the foundation. The foundation also has other programs supporting scholarship in athletic training. To learn more about the foundation, visit their website at http://www.natafoundation.org.

The most important supporters of scholarship in athletic training should be athletic trainers. Encouraging students to adopt scholarly approaches to the profession is paramount. This encouragement should come in clinical and classroom settings. A few suggested activities include[1]:

- Assigning students to read overviews of scholarship, preferably by a number of different authors
- Involving students as research assistants to faculty and graduate students
- Helping students understand the scientific method of problem solving. This will not only introduce them to scholarship but help sharpen their athletic training skills
- Teaching students how to read and interpret journal articles and then require them to do both
- Encouraging students to attend the free communication sessions at conferences
- Introducing the concepts of manuscript construction and requiring students to write papers in that style (I suggest the American Medical Association [AMA] style, since most journals in our profession use this style)
- Encouraging students to write for the *Journal of Athletic Training* Student Writing Contest
- Including critical thinking skills in all classes and clinical assignments
- Having students take a class in research methods
- Conducting original research as a project or a thesis

See Chapter Ten for more suggestions on teaching students about research.

Developing scholars and scholarly practitioners is essential to the health of our profession. A scholarly approach to the profession enhances the knowledge base in the profession, which improves patient care. Patients expect responsible practitioners to continually develop new ways to enhance and restore their health. We have to keep up our end of the deal.

REFERENCES

1. Knight KL, Ingersoll CD. Developing scholarship in athletic training. *Journal of Athletic Training*. 1998;33:271-274.

2. Delforge GD. Athletic training: a profession? Presented at the National Athletic Trainers' Association Annual Meeting and Clinical Symposia; June 1983; Denver, Colo.

3. Knight KL. Research in athletic training: a frill or a necessity? *Athl Train, JNATA*. 1988;23:212.

4. Osternig LR. Research in athletic training: the missing ingredient. *Athl Train, JNATA*. 1988;23:223-225.

5. Knight KL. Expanding our body of knowledge. *Athl Train, JNATA*. 1990;25:8.

6. Office of Research. *A Model for Directing Scholarly Work at Brigham Young University*. Provo, Utah: Brigham Young University; 1994.

7. Van Dalen DB. *Understanding Education Research*. 3rd ed. New York: McGraw-Hill Book Co; 1983:1-12.

8. Barry VE. *Invitation to Critical Thinking*. New York: CBS Publishing; 1984:181-183.

9. Wiersma W. *Research Methods in Education: An Introduction*. 4th ed. Boston, Mass: Allyn Bacon, Inc; 1986:17-19.

10. Mosey AC. The competent scholar. *Am J Occup Ther*. 1998;52:760-764.

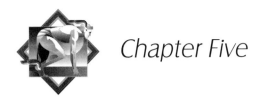

Chapter Five

Basics of Developing a Research Project

"Restlessness and discontent are the first necessities of progress." —*Thomas A. Edison*

Performing research is like any other professional task one undertakes: it must be well planned. Breaking the task into smaller pieces helps during the planning process. Developing a research project involves four major steps:

1. Developing the problem
2. Defining the problem
3. Formulating methods
4. Analyzing and interpreting results

It is not the scope of this text to fully explain all of these areas but to share some basic information and suggestions.

DEVELOPING THE PROBLEM

Development of a problem often stems from a clinical question. What do parents think of athletic training services in the high school setting? Can I get the same thermal effects from ultrasound using ultrasonic gel and a gel pad? Is there more cervical spine movement with the log roll or the lift and slide technique? And so on. Answering these questions helps us provide better patient care.

The first step in developing the problem is to ask questions like the ones above. Once you have an idea of the topic you'd like to investigate, you need to find out what is already known in that area. Reviewing the literature does this. Sometimes, the very question you are asking has already been asked and answered. Many times it has not, but there is some information relating to your question. You need to find out as much as you can about the topic so you can clearly define the problem later.

Reviewing the literature begins with what used to be called library work. Today we call it electronic database searches. Locating all pertinent articles in the area is the goal. Some electronic databases that may be pertinent to athletic training research include:

- MEDLINE
- Sport Discus
- ERIC
- PsycInfo
- ProQuest

College and university libraries include these and other databases. MEDLINE is available free on the web (http://www.nlm.nih.gov/databases/freemedl.html). Note: MEDLINE does not index some journals pertinent to athletic training, such as the *Journal of Athletic Training, Journal of Sport Rehabilitation*, and *Athletic Therapy Today*.

Once you locate articles pertinent to your question: read, read, read. Become familiar with all of the issues surrounding the topic. You will do a much better job of defining the problem if you are aware of all the pertinent literature. Organizing your information and your thoughts on the information is important. Making notecards can do this.

Notecards used to mean writing notes on 3" x 5" notecards. Details of the articles were included, such as bibliographic information for the paper, purpose of the study, notes about the methods, synopsis of the results, and conclusions. Notecards tend to be very personal. Each person would write down specific information to help him or her remember important aspects of the paper. Notecards worked well in their day, but too much time is spent physically writing the information on the card, and searching through the cards for specific information can become rather cumbersome.

Using electronic notecards is more efficient and effective. Electronic notecards do not necessarily need to be notecards at all. They can be in a database or just copied into a word processor document, depending on your computer savvy. Electronic database searches allow you to download the information about the articles you locate. The information will look something like the example in Table 5-1.

Abstracts may or may not be included, though I suggest saving as much information as you can. You can then add your notes to this entry. If placed in a word processing file, you can then do electronic searches within the document to find wanted information using the find function. This makes it much quicker to find papers that address specific topics than thumbing through actual notecards, and typed notes can be block copied into the manuscript as you are writing. Downloaded information from MEDLINE and other databases can also be imported into reference management software such as EndNotes (ISI ResearchSoft, Berkeley, Calif).

You may also wish to use the grid approach for literature review. This may be done in addition to or instead of the method described above. The grid can be developed in a spreadsheet or database, or by using the table function in a word processor. The grid includes pertinent information about the papers that you review. Information such as the author(s) name(s), date, independent variable, dependent variable, results, and comments may be included (Table 5-2). This method often requires hand-entry of information but is very helpful in organizing thoughts.

DEFINING THE PROBLEM

Once you have developed your problem, you must specifically define it. To do this, I suggest asking and answering the following questions:
- What is/are your research question(s)?
- What are your experimental hypotheses?
- What assumptions are you making?
- What are the delimitations in the study?
- Are there any limitations in the study?
- What are some important operational definitions in the study?
- What is the significance of the study?

What is/are Your Research Question(s)?

Ask yourself what you want to find out. For example, "Does ultrasound preceded by a hot pack improve range of motion more than ultrasound alone?" Research questions should be in the form of a question. Many of my students over the years have done a good job stating the purpose of their studies when asked this question. Before you can have a purpose for a study, however, you need to have a question to answer. You may have more than one question for a single study.

Table 5-1

EXAMPLE OF JOURNAL ARTICLE INFORMATION DOWNLOADED FROM MEDLINE

1: *Arch Phys Med Rehabil.* 2000 Sep;81(9):1199-203

Changes in soleus motoneuron pool excitability after artificial knee joint effusion.

Hopkins JT, Ingersoll CD, Edwards JE, Cordova ML

Athletic Training Department, Indiana State University, Terre Haute 47809, USA.

OBJECTIVE: To compare changes in the magnitude of soleus motoneuron excitability before and over a 4-hour period following artificial knee effusion. DESIGN: Before-after trial. SETTING: All measurements were collected in the Sports Injury Research Laboratory, Indiana State University. PARTICIPANTS: Eleven healthy and neurologically sound volunteers (mean age +/- SD, 24 +/- 3yr; height, 173.2 +/- 9.6cm; weight, 72.9 +/- 8.7kg) with no history of lower-extremity surgery and no lower extremity pathology in the last year. INTERVENTIONS: An area superolateral to the patella was cleaned and injected subcutaneously with 2mL of lidocaine for anesthetic purposes. With a second disposable syringe, 25mL of sterile saline was injected through the superolateral knee joint capsule into the joint space to mimic mechanical joint effusion. MAIN OUTCOME MEASURE: Hoffmann's reflex (H-reflex) was elicited by applying a percutaneous stimulus to the tibial nerve in the popliteal fossa. Seven to 12 stimuli were delivered at 20-second intervals with varying intensities to find the maximal H-reflex. The maximal H-reflex was measured five times at the same stimulus intensity with 20-second rest intervals. This measurement was recorded before injection and at 1-hour intervals following the injection for 4 hours. RESULTS: An overall difference between groups was found. Measurements from hours 3 and 4 were significantly higher than the preinjection measurements ($p < $ or $= .05$). CONCLUSIONS: The soleus motoneuron pool was not inhibited as expected. The soleus was facilitated beyond the preinjection level, showing that the quadriceps and soleus do not respond in the same way to artificial knee effusion. Because the quadriceps are normally inhibited during knee effusion, this facilitation could be the result of a compensatory reaction by the soleus in response to inhibited quadriceps. Further studies must be performed to determine the extent and duration of soleus motoneuron pool excitability in relation to quadriceps inhibition elicited by artificial knee effusion.

Publication Types:

  • Clinical trial

PMID: 10987162

Reprinted from Hopkins JT, Ingersoll CD, Edwards JE, Cordova ML. Changes in soleus motoneuron pool excitability after artificial knee joint effusion. Arch Phys Med Rehabil. 2000;81(9):1199-1203, with permission of Christopher D. Ingersoll.

Table 5-2				
THE GRID METHOD FOR LITERATURE REVIEWS				
Author(s)	Date	Independent Variables	Dependent Variables	Results
Jones, et al	1999	Ultrasound (US) coupling medium	Muscle temperature	"Super" gel does not result in increased temperature compared to regular gel
Smith	2000	US coupling medium	Muscle temperature	Gel pad results in the same temperature as "super" gel

What are Your Experimental Hypotheses?

Experimental (or research) hypotheses are statements of what you think is going to happen in your study. Null hypotheses are statements in the null form used primarily to establish the statistical comparisons to be made. Null hypotheses are important for statistical purposes but do little to help the investigator understand the literature and, hence, where their study fits into the big picture. Experimental hypotheses allow investigators to use their best judgment after reading the literature as to what might happen in the experiment. Sometimes, experimental hypotheses are the same as null hypotheses; however, a specific reason must be provided as to why treatments may be the same. If you are unable to state experimental hypotheses, there may not be enough information in the literature to justify your question or you may not have read extensively enough. See Table 5-3 for examples of experimental and null hypotheses.

What Assumptions are You Making?

Think carefully about any assumptions you are making. Some are easy. For example, we often assume that subjects are answering questions on a survey truthfully, but we have no way of knowing whether this assumption is true or not. Sometimes we can actually take measurements to determine whether an assumption is correct or not. For example, questions can be added into questionnaires to determine if subjects are being dishonest. Most of the time, it is impossible to tell and it has to remain an assumption.

We often assume that subjects are following directions. Sometimes they do not, but we must assume that they do or find a way to determine whether they have or not. In general, it is better to measure and know than to assume. You must start by writing down all of the assumptions you can think of.

What are the Delimitations in the Study?

Delimitations are choices you make in your study in order to make it workable. Choices are often made as to the type of subjects, treatments, or measuring systems used; these are delimitations. Delimitations in a study affect the extent to which the results of a study can be generalized. For example, a study evaluating postural control before a fall in elderly subjects may not be applicable to

Table 5-3

EXAMPLES OF EXPERIMENTAL AND NULL HYPOTHESIS STATEMENTS

Experimental Hypothesis	Null Hypothesis
Subjects wearing a lace-up ankle brace will have a higher vertical jump than subjects with taped ankles.	Vertical jump will be the same for subjects wearing a lace-up ankle brace and subjects with taped ankles.
Motoneuron pool recruitment following knee effusion will be greater using cryotherapy than transcutaneous electrical nerve stimulation (TENS) or no treatment.	Motoneuron pool recruitment following knee effusion will be the same whether using cryotherapy, TENS, or no treatment.

teenaged gymnasts. All studies have delimitations. It is important to identify them so that appropriate conclusions can be drawn and generalized.

Are There Any Limitations in the Study?

Limitations are shortcomings in the study. These are generally design flaws or other factors that severely limit the generalizability of the study. If you identify any of these at the beginning of the study, they should be rectified. Often, limitations are found after the study has been completed. Factors that the investigator did not consider at the beginning of the study are later found to have negatively affected the outcome. Much thought should be put into considering possible limitations. Finding limitations at the end of the study that could have been identified at the beginning with some thought is very frustrating and counterproductive.

What are Some Important Operational Definitions in the Study?

An operational definition is simply how you define a variable or term in your study. Operational definitions are important to help clarify what you mean when you use certain terms. Often, terms used in the literature have different meanings in different studies. While it is not important to list all operational definitions in a paper, it is helpful to provide them, as appropriate, in the text. In theses and in dissertations, an actual list of operational definitions is often required to help students clarify the meaning of terms.

What is the Significance of the Study?

Perhaps the most important step in defining the problem is to ask the "so what" question. If you carry out the experiment, what will it contribute to the literature? Importance does not necessarily mean immediate clinical application, but it should help enhance our understanding of issues fundamental to the profession.

FORMULATING METHODS

The methods of a study are the blueprint for how the study is to be conducted. Methods are often considered in five parts:

1. Research design
2. Subjects
3. Instruments
4. Procedures
5. Statistical analysis

Each of these areas is much more involved than described here, but I have tried to present some of the more critical issues for each area.

Selecting a Research Design

Research designs may be divided into four basic types: pre-experimental designs, true experimental designs, quasi-experimental designs, and other types of quasidesigns.[1] Each is used for specific situations and has unique advantages and disadvantages.

A special form of notation is often used to visualize research designs. Table 5-4 describes each symbol and its meaning.

PRE-EXPERIMENTAL DESIGNS

Pre-experimental designs control very few sources of invalidity; therefore, they are infrequently used. There are three basic types of pre-experimental designs: one-shot study, one-group pretest-posttest design, and static group comparison (see Table 5-5 for design notation). None of the three control for many sources of invalidity and none include random assignment of subjects into groups.

TRUE EXPERIMENTAL DESIGNS

True experimental designs are characterized by random formation of groups and maximal control of sources of invalidity. There are three types of experimental designs: randomized groups, pretest-posttest randomized groups, and the Solomon four-group design.

The randomized groups design involves random assignment of subjects into groups, one or more treatments, and posttest measurements. The simplest form includes a treatment group and a control group (see Table 5-5). More than one treatment group can be included and would be noted as a new line with subscripted Ts to denote multiple treatments. Although there is a practical limit to the number of treatment groups one might include, the number is not restricted.

The pretest-posttest randomized groups design is essentially the same as a randomized groups design except a pretest is included. As with the randomized groups design, there is no limit to the number of treatment groups that can be included. Including a pretest allows group comparisons before the intervention but also introduces possible learning of the measurement instrument.

The Solomon four-group design is designed to incorporate the advantages of both the randomized groups design and the pretest-posttest randomized groups design. All subjects are randomly assigned to groups but only half receive pretests or treatments. This design is specifically used if there is concern that pretests are affecting posttest measures.

QUASI-EXPERIMENTAL DESIGNS

Quasi-experimental designs are used in real-world settings. While they do not control as many factors as true experimental designs, they tend to be more generalized. The four major types include time series designs, reversal designs, nonequivalent control group designs, and ex post facto designs.

Time series designs include only one group. Multiple measurements are taken before a treatment is introduced, then multiple measurements are taken after the treatment. Four measurements are shown

Table 5-4

EXPERIMENTAL DESIGN NOTATION

Symbol	Meaning
R	Random assignment of subjects into groups.
O	Observation, measurement, or test. Subscripted numbers may be used to denote order.
T	Treatment or intervention. Subscripted numbers may be used to denote multiple administrations of the same treatment if on the same line or administration of different treatments if on different lines. Left blank for control groups.
--------	Represents intact groups if placed between groups.

Table 5-5

NOTATION FOR RESEARCH DESIGNS

Design	Notation
Pre-experimental	
One-shot study	$T \ O$
One-group pretest-posttest design	$O_1 \ T \ O_2$
Static group comparison	$T \quad O_1$ --------- O_2
True experimental	
Randomized groups design	$R \ T \ O_1$ $R \quad O_2$
Pretest-posttest randomized groups design	$R \ O_1 \ T \quad O_2$ $R \ O_3 \quad O_4$
Solomon four-group design	$R \ O_1 \ T \quad O_2$ $R \ O_3 \quad O_4$ $R \quad T \quad O_5$ $R \quad O_6$
Quasi-experimental	
Time series design	$O_1 \ O_2 \ O_3 \ O_4 \ T \quad O_5 \ O_6 \ O_7 \ O_8$
Reversal design	$O_1 \ O_2 \ T_1 \ O_3 \ O_4 \ T_2 \ O_5 \ O_6$

Table 5-5 (Continued)	
Design	**Notation**
Nonequivalent control group design	O_1 T O_2

	O_3 O_4
Ex post facto design	Same as static group comparison except treatment is not controlled by experimenter

before and after the treatment in Table 5-5, but it could be any number. Means of pretest and posttest scores can be compared to evaluate the effectiveness of the treatment.

Reversal designs also include a single group and multiple measurements before and after treatments. More than one treatment is introduced in a reversal design. Two measurements before and after treatments and two treatments are presented in Table 5-5, but any number could be used. Cumulative effects of treatments can be evaluated.

The nonequivalent control group design is similar to the randomized groups design, which is a true experimental design, except subjects are not randomly assigned to groups. Use of intact groups is sometimes necessary in real-world situations.

The ex post facto design is similar to the static group comparison design, which is a pre-experimental design, except the investigator has no control over the treatment. Treatments outside the control of the investigator may include characteristics such as gender, fitness level, or skill level. These characteristics are inherent in the subject before the experiment and cannot be (easily) changed.

OTHER DESIGNS

There are other research designs that are applicable to athletic training research but do not necessarily fit into the categories described. They include switched replication designs, epidemiological designs, and single subject designs.

Deciding on Subject Characteristics

Selecting subjects for your study is critical. Much of the research performed by athletic trainers has involved use of normal subjects. While research with normal subjects may provide some insight into the effectiveness of the interventions that we provide, it usually does not. Selecting subject characteristics determines the generalizability of your study. If you study children, it may be difficult to generalize to adults. If you use sedentary subjects, it is sometimes difficult to generalize to competitive athletes.

Considerations should be made in terms of both inclusion and exclusion factors. Inclusion factors may include things such as a mechanically unstable ankle, grade III concussion, or VO_2 above 50 ml/kg/sec. Exclusion criteria may include things such as an allergy to certain medications, recent surgery to the lower extremities, or previous exposure to cryotherapy.

All subjects should be volunteers and should be treated with dignity and respect. See Chapter Seven for more on protection of human subjects.

Selecting Instruments

Do your homework to make sure the instrument you are using is appropriate for what you are trying to measure. Just because an instrument can give you a number does not necessarily mean it is meaningful. Use the literature as a guide for finding instruments. For example, an instrument for measuring pain may be appropriate in certain circumstances but not in others.

Procedure

The procedure for an experiment is simply a step-by-step explanation of what was done. Every step in the procedure should be analyzed to make sure that the integrity of the experiment was not disrupted. Doing pilot work before beginning an experiment is very important. Pilot work helps identify unexpected problems, helps the investigator become proficient at using the instrument, and provides preliminary data that may be useful in determining things such as how many supplies to order, how many subjects will need to be recruited to have sufficient power to run your statistical analysis, etc. There are three important steps for developing procedures:
1. Do pilot work
2. Do more pilot work
3. Do even more pilot work if necessary

Finding problems or flaws in your procedure once you have started your experiment can be devastating. Find these problems before you start.

Carefully and accurately describing your procedure in writing is important for preparation of your manuscript but also to help remind you of all the things that must be done. I suggest developing a bulleted list of things that need to be done each time a subject is tested.

Statistical Analysis

Well, we finally got to the part most people dread. Most athletic trainers who express a fear or dislike for research attribute it to statistics. They view statistics as complex mathematical exercises for Mensa members. The amount of mathematics preparation needed to correctly select and interpret statistical tests is actually minimal. Addition, subtraction, multiplication, division, and exponentiation are the only math skills needed. Those skills are only necessary if you want to do the analyses by hand. Usually, we use computer software for that task.

The most important characteristic to have as a good statistician is logic. That being said, selecting the correct statistical analysis can sometimes be complex. Having taught statistics to graduate students for a number of years, I developed a table to provide guidance in selecting statistical analyses for their theses or research projects (Table 5-6). While this table does not address the minutia sometimes involved in choosing between related tests, it typically helps students at least find the right classification of analyses. The scope of this text is not to provide indepth descriptions for statistical analyses. Please refer to the recommended reading section for texts that do.

ANALYZING AND INTERPRETING RESULTS

As previously stated, statistical analyses are typically done with a computer. Several software packages exist for this purpose. Statistical Package for the Social Sciences ([SPSS] SPSS Inc, Chicago, IL), Statistical Analysis Software ([SAS] SAS Inc, Cary, NC), and Minitab (Minitab Inc., State College, PA) are among the more popular packages.

Reporting the outcome of the statistical tests is important (see Chapter Eight about presenting results in a manuscript), but interpreting the meaning of these outcomes is more important; ie, explaining what the results mean is the more important task. This is how a theory is built (see Chapter Four

Table 5-6

GUIDELINES FOR SELECTING A STATISTICAL TEST*

Test	# DVs	# IVs	# Levels IV	Ss do all Tx?	Data Distribution	Test Statistic	Ho
Independent t-test	1	1	2	No	Normal	t	$\mu_1 = \mu_2$
Dependent t-test	1	1	2	Yes	Normal	t	$\mu_1 = \mu_2$
One-way analysis of variance (ANOVA)	1	1	>2	No	Normal	F	$\mu_1 = \mu_2 = \ldots = \mu_k$
One-way repeated measures ANOVA	1	1	>2	Yes	Normal	F	$\mu_1 = \mu_2 = \ldots = \mu_k$
Two-way ANOVA	1	2	2 or >	No	Normal	F	$\mu_{11} = \mu_{12} = \ldots = \mu_{1k}$ $\mu_{21} = \mu_{22} = \ldots = \mu_{2k}$
Two-way repeated measures ANOVA‡	1	2	2 or >	Yes	Normal	F	$\mu_{11} = \mu_{12} = \ldots = \mu_{1k}$ $\mu_{21} = \mu_{22} = \ldots = \mu_{2k}$
k-way ANOVA	1	j	2 or >	No	Normal	F	$\mu_{11} = \mu_{12} = \ldots = \mu_{1k}$ $\mu_{21} = \mu_{22} = \ldots = \mu_{2k}$ $\mu_{j1} = \mu_{j2} = \ldots = \mu_{jk}$
k-way repeated measures ANOVA‡	1	j	2 or >	Yes	Normal	F	$\mu_{11} = \mu_{12} = \ldots = \mu_{1k}$ $\mu_{21} = \mu_{22} = \ldots = \mu_{2k}$ $\mu_{j1} = \mu_{j2} = \ldots = \mu_{jk}$
Hotelling's T^2	j	1	2	Yes/No	Normal	T^2	†
One-way multivariate analysis of variance (MANOVA)	j	1	> 2	No	Normal	Λ	†

Table 5-6 (Continued)

Test	# DVs	# IVs	# Levels IV	Ss do all Tx?	Data Distribution	Test Statistic	Ho
One-way repeated measures MANOVA‡	j	1	>2	Yes	Normal	¥	†
Two-way MANOVA	j	2	2 or >	No	Normal	¥	†
Two-way repeated measures MANOVA‡	j	2	2 or >	Yes	Normal	¥	†
k-way MANOVA	j	j	2 or >	No	Normal	¥	†
k-way repeated measures MANOVA‡	j	j	2 or >	Yes	Normal	¥	†
Mann-Whitney U test	1	1	2	No	Not normal	U	$\mu_1 = \mu_2$
Wilcoxon matched-pairs signed-rank test	1	1	2	Yes	Not normal	T	$\mu_1 = \mu_2$
Kruskal-Wallis test	1	1	>2	No	Not normal	H	$\mu_1 = \mu_2 = \ldots = \mu_k$
Friedman test	1	j	2 or >	Yes	Not normal	χ^2	$\mu_{11} = \mu_{12} = \ldots = \mu_{1k}$ $\mu_{21} = \mu_{22} = \ldots = \mu_{2k}$ $\mu_{j1} = \mu_{j2} = \ldots = \mu_{jk}$

*Not all statistical tests are included in this table; DV = dependent variable; IV = independent variable; Ss do all tx = all subjects do treatments; Ho = null hypothesis; j = number greater than 2; ¥ = there are several multivariate test statistics; Wilk's λ and Roy's Largest Root are among the more popular; † = a topic for another day (need to discuss matrices first); ‡ = mixed models are also possible in which some factors have repeated measures and some do not for more on the importance of building a theory). Putting your results in context with what others have found allows the continued development of theory. Communicating the interpretation of your results also helps clinicians reading your manuscript put them into action helping patients.

REFERENCE

1. Thomas JR, Nelson JK. *Research Methods in Physical Activity.* 3rd ed. Champaign, Ill: Human Kinetics; 1996:351-363.

RECOMMENDED READING

Ackerman WB, Lohnes PR. *Research Methods for Nurses.* New York: McGraw-Hill; 1981.

Bailey DM. *Research for the Health Professional: A Practical Guide.* 2nd ed. Philadelphia, Pa: FA Davis; 1997.

Bell FD. *Basic Biostatistics: Concepts for the Health Sciences.* Dubuque, Iowa: Wm C Brown Publishers; 1995.

Berg BL. *Qualitative Research Methods for the Social Sciences.* 2nd ed. Boston, Mass: Allyn and Bacon; 1995.

Bernard HR. *Research Methods in Anthropology: Qualitative and Quantitative Approaches.* Thousand Oaks, Calif: Sage Publications; 1994.

Brodie DA, Williams JG, Owens RG. *Research Methods for the Health Sciences.* New York: Harwood Academic Publishers; 1994.

Conover WJ. *Practical Nonparametric Statistics.* 2nd ed. New York: John Wiley & Sons; 1980.

Daniel WW. *Biostatistics: A Foundation for Analysis in the Health Sciences.* 5th ed. New York: John Wiley & Sons; 1991.

Everitt B. *The Cambridge Dictionary of Statistics.* Cambridge, UK: Cambridge University Press; 1998.

Fisher L, van Belle G. *Biostatistics: A Methodology for the Health Sciences.* New York: John Wiley & Sons; 1993.

Graziano AM, Raulin ML. *Research Methods: A Process of Inquiry.* New York: Harper & Row; 1989.

Nachmias D, Nachmias C. *Research Methods in the Social Sciences.* New York: St. Martin's Press; 1976.

Neutens JJ, Rubinson L. *Research Techniques for the Health Sciences.* 2nd ed. Boston, Mass: Allyn and Bacon; 1997.

Sahai H, Khurshid A. *Statistics in Epidemiology: Methods, Techniques, and Applications.* Boca Raton, Fla: CRC Press; 1996.

Shelley SI. *Research Methods in Nursing and Health.* Boston, Mass: Little, Brown and Co; 1984.

Shott S. *Statistics for Health Professionals.* Philadelphia, Pa: WB Saunders; 1990.

Stevens J. *Applied Multivariate Statistics for the Social Sciences.* Hillsdale, NJ: Lawrence Erlbaum Associates; 1986.

Vincent WJ. *Statistics in Kinesiology.* 2nd ed. Champaign, Ill: Human Kinetics; 1999.

Walizer MH, Wienir PL. *Research Methods and Analysis: Searching for Relationships.* New York: Harper & Row; 1978.

Wassertheil-Smoller S. *Biostatistics and Epidemiology: A Primer for Health Professionals.* 2nd ed. New York: Springer-Verlag; 1995.

Wiersma W. *Research Methods in Education: An Introduction.* 6th ed. Boston, Mass: Allyn and Bacon; 1995.

Zolman JF. *Biostatistics: Experimental Design and Statistical Inference.* New York: Oxford University Press; 1993.

Chapter Six

The Athletic Trainer
as a Researcher

"The whole of science is nothing more than a refinement of everyday thinking." —Albert Einstein

Athletic trainers behave like researchers every day. Many of the clinical tools we have developed are similar to processes of the scientific method. The biggest challenges are some of the more formalized processes of research, such as selection of correct research designs and statistical analyses. With some help and knowledge, these processes can be conquered. Building a research network for athletic trainers will help bring the necessary resources together so everyone can contribute to the athletic training knowledge base.

ATHLETIC TRAINING PRACTICE AND THE SCIENTIFIC METHOD

The scientific method is very much like a situation in which you are evaluating an injury:
1. Develop the problem (take a history)
2. Formulate a hypothesis (what you think is wrong)
3. Gather data (do special tests)
4. Analyze and interpret the results (determine what is wrong based on the results of the tests)

Doing research is simply formalizing a process that we practice every day. The difference between research and what we do every day is that during a research project we support and document what we do more extensively.

When developing a research problem, we draw extensively upon the literature to know what has been done already. We may refer to a reference when taking a history during an injury evaluation, but more often we depend on what we have already learned.

Formulating a hypothesis during a research project is just a formalized version of what we do as we work through a differential diagnosis during the evaluation process. We are trying to determine what is happening or what is wrong. In research, we use hypotheses to develop research designs and select statistical analyses. Deciding which research designs or statistical analyses to use for a specific study draws on the same learning process we have already developed for determining which special test to use to ascertain the type of injury incurred. Just as we might decide to use the Lachman's test to evaluate a possible ACL injury, we can decide to use a pretest-posttest randomized groups design or repeated measures ANOVA.

Collecting data during a research project is much the same as performing the tests done during an injury evaluation. Great lengths are taken to collect the information in a specific way to ensure its accuracy so appropriate conclusions can be drawn. The data are recorded so they can be analyzed later. Special pieces of equipment are often used to collect information about the subject's/patient's ability to perform a specific task. Data collection is one of the most time-consuming processes in research.

Because it can fit well into processes that occur every day in athletic training practice, data can often be collected without a lot of extra work.

We analyze and interpret results every day. Clinically, we make decisions based on the evaluations we perform. In research we use statistical analyses to assist with our decisions. Essentially, we are computing mathematical probabilities before stating what we think is happening in research. Once we state what we think is happening, we need to attempt to explain why we think the injury or research results turned out the way they did. Clinically, we may draw upon the literature, but most often we draw upon our experience. In research, we certainly draw upon our past experiences, but we also draw heavily on others' experiences as well (eg, we compare our results to those in the literature). We try to determine where our results fit into the big picture. This contributes to the advancement of theory, which in turn enhances our understanding of what we hope is the truth. Finally, we draw conclusions both clinically and in a research report. Our conclusions should be based on our findings regardless of the setting.

Research requires refinement of tools we already possess. In fact, development of research skills improves clinical decision-making abilities. The ability to perform research and ultimately share it (presentation or publication) allows us to share our knowledge and improve the clinical practices of all athletic trainers.

RESEARCH DESIGN AND STATISTICS: THE CURSE?

I have not met a person yet who understands everything there is to know about statistics or research design. I have met a few who know quite a bit, but most have a functional knowledge of the aspects of statistics or research designs that affect them the most.

I have not met a person yet who understands everything there is to know about athletic training. I have met a few who know quite a bit, but most have a functional knowledge of the aspects of athletic training that affect them the most.

Do not be intimidated by research design and statistics. I do not intend to underestimate the complexity of some research designs or the important subtleties of specific statistical analyses; however, most research designs are quite straightforward. Many statistical analyses are rather simple to understand and execute. Think of it as a game with rules: learn the rules, win the game. There are lots of places to get help (see the Building an Athletic Training Research Network section later in this chapter). It is okay to get help. Some of my favorite research projects were those in which I collaborated with colleagues who had a good idea but were not sure about research design or statistics and asked for help.

Now that I have hopefully, at least partially, convinced you to not be intimidated by research design and statistics, I want to say, "Do not underestimate the importance of research design and statistics." Improper design will prevent testing of the intended hypothesis and improper statistical analyses will not allow proper conclusions to be drawn.

HOW TO GET INVOLVED IN RESEARCH

There are numerous ways athletic trainers can become involved in research:
- Get involved in others' research
- Develop or join a research network (see Building an Athletic Training Research Network later in this chapter)
- Get your physician(s) involved in your research or become involved in theirs
- Work research into your everyday practice (remember, you are collecting data every day)
- Develop your own research project and assemble a team to tackle your question
- Write a grant to fund your research (see Chapter Nine)

BUILDING AN ATHLETIC TRAINING RESEARCH NETWORK

In order for people who are interested in performing research to find either people who have similar interests or people who have specific research skills, a medium must be developed to allow these interactions. I think a web page could be developed to meet this need. This web page could serve as a "collaboratory." Collaboratories have been built by other professionals.[1,2]

In order for athletic trainers to collaborate on research, they need the following in their collaboratory:

- Find out who else has similar interests
- Find experts in the area and statistical and research design help
- A way to "get together" to refine their ideas, state hypotheses, work out methods, develop proposals, write grants for funding, etc
- Divide responsibilities for the research project
- A way to share data
- A way to share documents relevant to the research (ie, the manuscript, statistical output, data files, etc)

REFERENCES

1. Hanak T, Hoang B, Boucher B, Keely G. The development of a web page to promote clinicians' and students' collaboration in research. *J Allied Health*. 1999;28:252-256.

2. Physical therapy research partnership: a database of current research ideas and contacts. Available at: http://pages.hotbot.com/health/ptrp. Accessed July 22, 2000.

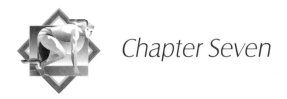

Chapter Seven

Protecting Human Subjects

"The voluntary consent of the human subject is absolutely essential." —The Nuremberg Code

Athletic training research often involves using human subjects. The people who volunteer to participate in athletic training research sometimes realize the direct benefits of their participation (eg, a new treatment that allows faster rehabilitation), but they also assume risk. The balance between risks and benefits must be carefully considered before asking humans to participate in your research project.

A large percentage of current research in athletic training is performed on normal subjects (ie, those without conditions, injuries, illnesses, etc). While individuals who are ill or injured benefit from experimental treatments, normal subjects often do not. They do consent to participate as subjects, however. We have a duty to minimize the risks presented to these subjects and maximize the benefits to the knowledge base.

HISTORY OF THE PROTECTION OF HUMAN RESEARCH SUBJECTS

Policies for the use of humans as research subjects began following World War II. Attempts were made to prevent the types of experiments that Nazi doctors carried out on war prisoners. The Nuremberg Code[1] (Table 7-1), written for use in the military tribunal that convened to bring the doctors to trial, established the concept that in research "the voluntary consent of the human subject is absolutely essential." This precept has remained basic to policies concerning human subjects throughout its development.

Inappropriate treatment of human subjects in research continued even after the establishment of the Nuremberg Code. For example, in 1932, US Public Health Service doctors initiated a study ("the Tuskegee study") of poor African-American men who had syphilis. Even after penicillin was discovered as a cure in 1943, the researchers continued to observe the progression of the disease in these subjects without treating it. The men were not told they had syphilis or that there was a cure for their illness. Also, between 1944 and 1974, the US government sponsored nearly 4000 radiation experiments on humans.

In 1964, the World Medical Association developed the Declaration of Helsinki[2] (Table 7-2). This document stated that "the purpose of biomedical research involving human subjects must be to improve diagnostic, therapeutic, and prophylactic procedures, and the understanding of the aetiology and pathogenesis of disease." This basic sentiment is retained in more modern documents involving protection of human research subjects. The World Medical Association is in the process of revising the Declaration of Helsinki.

In 1974, the first US regulations for protecting human subjects became effective when policies adopted in 1966 by the National Institutes of Health (NIH) were raised to regulatory status. These

Table 7-1

THE NUREMBERG CODE

The voluntary consent of the human subject is absolutely essential. This means that the person involved should have legal capacity to give consent; should be so situated as to be able to exercise free power of choice without the intervention of any element of force, fraud, deceit, duress, over-reaching, or other ulterior form of constraint or coercion; and should have sufficient knowledge and comprehension of the elements of the subject matter involved as to enable him to make an understanding and enlightened decision. This latter element requires that before the acceptance of an affirmative decision by the experimental subject there should be made known to him the nature, duration, and purpose of the experiment; the method and means by which it is to be conducted; all inconveniences and hazards reasonably to be expected; and the effects upon his health or person which may possibly come from his participation in the experiment.

1. The duty and responsibility for ascertaining the quality of the consent rests upon each individual who initiates, directs, or engages in the experiment. It is a personal duty and responsibility which may not be delegated to another with impunity.

2. The experiment should be such as to yield fruitful results for the good of society, unprocurable by other methods or means of study, and not random and unnecessary in nature.

3. The experiment should be so designed and based on the results of animal experimentation and a knowledge of the natural history of the disease or other problem under study that the anticipated results will justify the performance of the experiment.

4. The experiment should be so conducted as to avoid all unnecessary physical and mental suffering and injury.

5. No experiment should be conducted where there is a prior reason to believe that death or disabling injury will occur; except, perhaps, in those experiments where the experimental physicians also serve as subjects.

6. The degree of risk to be taken should never exceed that determined by the humanitarian importance of the problem to be solved by the experiment.

7. Proper preparations should be made and adequate facilities provided to protect the experimental subject against even remote possibilities of injury, disability, or death.

8. The experiment should be conducted only by scientifically qualified persons. The highest degree of skill and care should be required through all stages of the experiment of those who conduct or engage in the experiment.

9. During the course of the experiment the human subject should be at liberty to bring the experiment to an end if he has reached the physical or mental state where continuation of the experiment seems to him to be impossible.

Table 7-1 (Continued)

10. During the course of the experiment the scientist in charge must be prepared to terminate the experiment at any stage, if he has probable cause to believe, in the exercise of the good faith, superior skill, and careful judgment required of him, that a continuation of the experiment is likely to result in injury, disability, or death to the experimental subject.

Table 7-2

THE DECLARATION OF HELSINKI

A. INTRODUCTION

1. The World Medical Association has developed the Declaration of Helsinki as a statement of ethical principles to provide guidance to physicians and other participants in medical research involving human subjects. Medical research involving human subjects includes research on identifiable human material or identifiable data.

2. It is the duty of the physician to promote and safeguard the health of the people. The physician's knowledge and conscience are dedicated to the fulfillment of this duty.

3. The Declaration of Geneva of the World Medical Association binds the physician with the words, "The health of my patient will be my first consideration," and the International Code of Medical Ethics declares that, "A physician shall act only in the patient's interest when providing medical care which might have the effect of weakening the physical and mental condition of the patient."

4. Medical progress is based on research which ultimately must rest in part on experimentation involving human subjects.

5. In medical research on human subjects, considerations related to the well-being of the human subject should take precedence over the interests of science and society.

6. The primary purpose of medical research involving human subjects is to improve prophylactic, diagnostic and therapeutic procedures and the understanding of the aetiology and pathogenesis of disease. Even the best proven prophylactic, diagnostic, and therapeutic methods must continuously be challenged through research for their effectiveness, efficiency, accessibility and quality.

7. In current medical practice and in medical research, most prophylactic, diagnostic and therapeutic procedures involve risks and burdens.

8. Medical research is subject to ethical standards that promote respect for all human beings and protect their health and rights. Some research populations are vulnerable and need special protection. The particular needs of the economically and medically disadvantaged must be recognized. Special attention is also required for those who cannot give or refuse consent for themselves, for those who may be subject to giving consent under duress, for those who will not benefit personally from the research and for those for whom the research is combined with care.

Table 7-2 (Continued)

9. Research Investigators should be aware of the ethical, legal and regulatory require-ments for research on human subjects in their own countries as well as applicable international requirements. No national ethical, legal or regulatory requirement should be allowed to reduce or eliminate any of the protections for human subjects set forth in this Declaration.

B. BASIC PRINCIPLES FOR ALL MEDICAL RESEARCH

10. It is the duty of the physician in medical research to protect the life, health, priva-cy, and dignity of the human subject.

11. Medical research involving human subjects must conform to generally accepted scientific principles, be based on a thorough knowledge of the scientific literature, other relevant sources of information, and on adequate laboratory and, where appropriate, animal experimentation.

12. Appropriate caution must be exercised in the conduct of research which may affect the environment, and the welfare of animals used for research must be respected.

13. The design and performance of each experimental procedure involving human subjects should be clearly formulated in an experimental protocol. This protocol should be submitted for consideration, comment, guidance, and where appropri-ate, approval to a specially appointed ethical review committee, which must be independent of the investigator, the sponsor or any other kind of undue influ-ence. This independent committee should be in conformity with the laws and reg-ulations of the country in which the research experiment is performed. The com-mittee has the right to monitor ongoing trials. The researcher has the obligation to provide monitoring information to the committee, especially any serious adverse events. The researcher should also submit to the committee, for review, information regarding funding, sponsors, institutional affiliations, other potential conflicts of interest and incentives for subjects.

14. The research protocol should always contain a statement of the ethical considera-tions involved and should indicate that there is compliance with the principles enunciated in this Declaration.

15. Medical research involving human subjects should be conducted only by scientifi-cally qualified persons and under the supervision of a clinically competent medical person. The responsibility for the human subject must always rest with a medical-ly qualified person and never rest on the subject of the research, even though the subject has given consent.

16. Every medical research project involving human subjects should be preceded by careful assessment of predictable risks and burdens in comparison with foresee-able benefits to the subject or to others. This does not preclude the participation of healthy volunteers in medical research. The design of all studies should be pub-licly available.

Table 7-2 (Continued)

17. Physicians should abstain from engaging in research projects involving human subjects unless they are confident that the risks involved have been adequately assessed and can be satisfactorily managed. Physicians should cease any investigation if the risks are found to outweigh the potential benefits or if there is conclusive proof of positive and beneficial results.

18. Medical research involving human subjects should only be conducted if the importance of the objective outweighs the inherent risks and burdens to the subject. This is especially important when the human subjects are healthy volunteers.

19. Medical research is only justified if there is a reasonable likelihood that the populations in which the research is carried out stand to benefit from the results of the research.

20. The subjects must be volunteers and informed participants in the research project.

21. The right of research subjects to safeguard their integrity must always be respected. Every precaution should be taken to respect the privacy of the subject, the confidentiality of the patient's information and to minimize the impact of the study on the subject's physical and mental integrity and on the personality of the subject.

22. In any research on human beings, each potential subject must be adequately informed of the aims, methods, sources of funding, any possible conflicts of interest, institutional affiliations of the researcher, the anticipated benefits and potential risks of the study and the discomfort it may entail. The subject should be informed of the right to abstain from participation in the study or to withdraw consent to participate at any time without reprisal. After ensuring that the subject has understood the information, the physician should then obtain the subject's freely-given informed consent, preferably in writing. If the consent cannot be obtained in writing, the non-written consent must be formally documented and witnessed.

23. When obtaining informed consent for the research project the physician should be particularly cautious if the subject is in a dependent relationship with the physician or may consent under duress. In that case the informed consent should be obtained by a well-informed physician who is not engaged in the investigation and who is completely independent of this relationship.

24. For a research subject who is legally incompetent, physically or mentally incapable of giving consent or is a legally incompetent minor, the investigator must obtain informed consent from the legally authorized representative in accordance with applicable law. These groups should not be included in research unless the research is necessary to promote the health of the population represented and this research cannot instead be performed on legally competent persons.

25. When a subject deemed legally incompetent, such as a minor child, is able to give assent to decisions about participation in research, the investigator must obtain that assent in addition to the consent of the legally authorized representative.

Table 7-2 (Continued)

26. Research on individuals from whom it is not possible to obtain consent, including proxy or advance consent, should be done only if the physical/mental condition that prevents obtaining informed consent is a necessary characteristic of the research population. The specific reasons for involving research subjects with a condition that renders them unable to give informed consent should be stated in the experimental protocol for consideration and approval of the review committee. The protocol should state that consent to remain in the research should be obtained as soon as possible from the individual or a legally authorized surrogate.

27. Both authors and publishers have ethical obligations. In publication of the results of research, the investigators are obliged to preserve the accuracy of the results. Negative as well as positive results should be published or otherwise publicly available. Sources of funding, institutional affiliations and any possible conflicts of interest should be declared in the publication. Reports of experimentation not in accordance with the principles laid down in this Declaration should not be accepted for publication.

C. ADDITIONAL PRINCIPLES FOR MEDICAL RESEARCH COMBINED WITH MEDICAL CARE

28. The physician may combine medical research with medical care, only to the extent that the research is justified by its potential prophylactic, diagnostic or therapeutic value. When medical research is combined with medical care, additional standards apply to protect the patients who are research subjects.

29. The benefits, risks, burdens and effectiveness of a new method should be tested against those of the best current prophylactic, diagnostic, and therapeutic methods. This does not exclude the use of placebo, or no treatment, in studies where no proven prophylactic, diagnostic or therapeutic method exists.

30. At the conclusion of the study, every patient entered into the study should be assured of access to the best proven prophylactic, diagnostic and therapeutic methods identified by the study.

31. The physician should fully inform the patient which aspects of the care are related to the research. The refusal of a patient to participate in a study must never interfere with the patient-physician relationship.

32. In the treatment of a patient, where proven prophylactic, diagnostic and therapeutic methods do not exist or have been ineffective, the physician, with informed consent from the patient, must be free to use unproven or new prophylactic, diagnostic and therapeutic measures, if in the physician's judgment it offers hope of saving life, re-establishing health or alleviating suffering. Where possible, these measures should be made the object of research, designed to evaluate their safety and efficacy. In all cases, new information should be recorded and, where appropriate, published. The other relevant guidelines of this Declaration should be followed.

regulations established the institutional review board (IRB) as a mechanism for safeguarding human participation in research. The IRB continues to be the primary mechanism by which experiments on human subjects are approved.

From 1974 to 1978, the National Commission for the Protection of Human Subjects in Biomedical and Behavioral Research met to define the ethical principles that govern research using human subjects and set guidelines for its conduct. The commission's report was titled *The Belmont Report*[3] (Table 7-3).

In 1981, regulations were added to the Code of Federal Regulations, Title 45 Part 46, and have since been revised twice, most recently on June 18, 1991. The 1991 revisions, also known as The Common Rule, were adopted by 16 federal agencies that support human subjects research.[4]

DEVELOPING AN INSTITUTIONAL REVIEW BOARD

One of the greatest challenges for athletic trainers attempting to do research in clinics or other parts of the private sector is the lack of an IRB. Many funding agencies (eg, the NATA Foundation) and journals (eg, the *Journal of Athletic Training*) require proof of IRB approval. Developing an IRB can be done anywhere by anyone as long as institutional recognition of the group is granted. *The Institutional Review Board Guidebook*[5] provides guidelines for development and operation of an IRB.

The Office for Protection from Research Risks produced a videotape series, entitled *Protecting Human Subjects,* that consists of three instructional videotapes:

1. "Evolving Concern: Protection for Human Subjects" traces the development of today's comprehensive program to protect human subjects of research from earlier ethical codes and societal concerns. This film selected historic events in behavioral and biomedical research to show why protection is needed and how it came about.
2. "Balancing Society's Mandates: Criteria for Protocol Review" depicts an IRB in action. Dr. Edmund Pellegrino, director of the Kennedy Institute of Ethics, explains the basis for the criteria that an IRB follows when reviewing research. In commenting on IRB deliberations, he points out why the IRB seeks clarification and information from the researcher.
3. "The Belmont Report: Basic Ethical Principles and Their Application" describes the basic ethical principles that underlie research involving human subjects: respect for persons, beneficence, and justice. This film illustrates their application in case studies of biomedical and behavioral research and shows the principles at work in the resolution of ethical conflicts.

These videotapes are free and can be ordered from Darlene Marie Ross, Education Coordinator, Office for Human Research Protections, 6100 Executive Blvd, Suite 3B01, Rockville, MD 20879 (301-435-5648 or FAX 301-402-4256). They should be mandatory viewing for research methods classes.

Table 7-3

THE BELMONT REPORT

AGENCY: Department of Health, Education, and Welfare.

ACTION: Notice of Report for Public Comment.

SUMMARY: On July 12, 1974, the National Research Act (Pub. L. 93-348) was signed into law, thereby creating the National Commission for the Protection of Human Subjects of Biomedical and Behavioral Research. One of the charges to the Commission was to identify the basic ethical principles that should underlie the conduct of biomedical and behavioral research involving human subjects and to develop guidelines which should be followed to assure that such research is conducted in accordance with those principles. In carrying out the above, the Commission was directed to consider: **(i)** the boundaries between biomedical and behavioral research and the accepted and routine practice of medicine, **(ii)** the role of assessment of risk-benefit criteria in the determination of the appropriateness of research involving human subjects, **(iii)** appropriate guidelines for the selection of human subjects for participation in such research and **(iv)** the nature and definition of informed consent in various research settings.

The Belmont Report attempts to summarize the basic ethical principles identified by the Commission in the course of its deliberations. It is the outgrowth of an intensive four-day period of discussions that were held in February 1976 at the Smithsonian Institution's Belmont Conference Center supplemented by the monthly deliberations of the Commission that were held over a period of nearly four years. It is a statement of basic ethical principles and guidelines that should assist in resolving the ethical problems that surround the conduct of research with human subjects. By publishing the Report in the Federal Register, and providing reprints upon request, the Secretary intends that it may be made readily available to scientists, members of Institutional Review Boards, and Federal employees. The two-volume Appendix, containing the lengthy reports of experts and specialists who assisted the Commission in fulfilling this part of its charge, is available as DHEW Publication No. (OS) 78-0013 and No. (OS) 78-0014, for sale by the Superintendent of Documents, U.S. Government Printing Office, Washington, D.C. 20402.

Unlike most other reports of the Commission, the Belmont Report does not make specific recommendations for administrative action by the Secretary of Health, Education, and Welfare. Rather, the Commission recommended that the Belmont Report be adopted in its entirety, as a statement of the Department's policy. The Department requests public comment on this recommendation.

Ethical Principles & Guidelines for Research Involving Human Subjects

Scientific research has produced substantial social benefits. It has also posed some troubling ethical questions. Public attention was drawn to these questions by reported abuses of human subjects in biomedical experiments, especially during the Second World War. During the Nuremberg War Crime Trials, the Nuremberg Code was drafted as a set of standards for judging physicians and scientists who had conducted biomedical experiments on concentration camp prisoners. This code became the prototype of many later codes (A) intended to assure that research involving human subjects would be carried out in an ethical manner.

Table 7-3 (Continued)

The codes consist of rules, some general, others specific, that guide the investigators or the reviewers of research in their work. Such rules often are inadequate to cover complex situations; at times they come into conflict, and they are frequently difficult to interpret or apply. Broader ethical principles will provide a basis on which specific rules may be formulated, criticized and interpreted.

Three principles, or general prescriptive judgments, that are relevant to research involving human subjects are identified in this statement. Other principles may also be relevant. These three are comprehensive, however, and are stated at a level of generalization that should assist scientists, subjects, reviewers and interested citizens to understand the ethical issues inherent in research involving human subjects. These principles cannot always be applied so as to resolve beyond dispute particular ethical problems. The objective is to provide an analytical framework that will guide the resolution of ethical problems arising from research involving human subjects.

This statement consists of a distinction between research and practice, a discussion of the three basic ethical principles, and remarks about the application of these principles.

Part A: Boundaries Between Practice and Research

A. Boundaries Between Practice and Research

It is important to distinguish between biomedical and behavioral research, on the one hand, and the practice of accepted therapy on the other, in order to know what activities ought to undergo review for the protection of human subjects of research. The distinction between research and practice is blurred partly because both often occur together (as in research designed to evaluate a therapy) and partly because notable departures from standard practice are often called "experimental" when the terms "experimental" and "research" are not carefully defined.

For the most part, the term "practice" refers to interventions that are designed solely to enhance the well-being of an individual patient or client and that have a reasonable expectation of success. The purpose of medical or behavioral practice is to provide diagnosis, preventive treatment or therapy to particular individuals (B). By contrast, the term "research" designates an activity designed to test a hypothesis, permit conclusions to be drawn, and thereby to develop or contribute to generalizable knowledge (expressed, for example, in theories, principles, and statements of relationships). Research is usually described in a formal protocol that sets forth an objective and a set of procedures designed to reach that objective.

When a clinician departs in a significant way from standard or accepted practice, the innovation does not, in and of itself, constitute research. The fact that a procedure is "experimental," in the sense of new, untested or different, does not automatically place it in the category of research. Radically new procedures of this description should, however, be made the object of formal research at an early stage in order to determine whether they are safe and effective. Thus, it is the responsibility of medical practice committees, for example, to insist that a major innovation be incorporated into a formal research project (C).

Table 7-3 (Continued)

Research and practice may be carried on together when research is designed to evaluate the safety and efficacy of a therapy. This need not cause any confusion regarding whether or not the activity requires review; the general rule is that if there is any element of research in an activity, that activity should undergo review for the protection of human subjects.

Part B: Basic Ethical Principles

B. Basic Ethical Principles

The expression "basic ethical principles" refers to those general judgments that serve as a basic justification for the many particular ethical prescriptions and evaluations of human actions. Three basic principles, among those generally accepted in our cultural tradition, are particularly relevant to the ethics of research involving human subjects: the principles of respect of persons, beneficence and justice.

1. Respect for Persons. Respect for persons incorporates at least two ethical convictions: first, that individuals should be treated as autonomous agents, and second, that persons with diminished autonomy are entitled to protection. The principle of respect for persons thus divides into two separate moral requirements: the requirement to acknowledge autonomy and the requirement to protect those with diminished autonomy.

An autonomous person is an individual capable of deliberation about personal goals and of acting under the direction of such deliberation. To respect autonomy is to give weight to autonomous persons' considered opinions and choices while refraining from obstructing their actions unless they are clearly detrimental to others. To show lack of respect for an autonomous agent is to repudiate that person's considered judgments, to deny an individual the freedom to act on those considered judgments, or to withhold information necessary to make a considered judgment, when there are no compelling reasons to do so.

However, not every human being is capable of self-determination. The capacity for self-determination matures during an individual's life, and some individuals lose this capacity wholly or in part because of illness, mental disability, or circumstances that severely restrict liberty. Respect for the immature and the incapacitated may require protecting them as they mature or while they are incapacitated.

Some persons are in need of extensive protection, even to the point of excluding them from activities which may harm them; other persons require little protection beyond making sure they undertake activities freely and with awareness of possible adverse consequence. The extent of protection afforded should depend upon the risk of harm and the likelihood of benefit. The judgment that any individual lacks autonomy should be periodically reevaluated and will vary in different situations.

In most cases of research involving human subjects, respect for persons demands that subjects enter into the research voluntarily and with adequate information. In some situations, however, application of the principle is not obvious. The involvement of prisoners as subjects of research provides an instructive example. On the one hand, it would seem that the principle of respect for persons requires that prisoners not be deprived of the opportunity to volunteer for research. On the other hand, under prison conditions they

Table 7-3 (Continued)

may be subtly coerced or unduly influenced to engage in research activities for which they would not otherwise volunteer. Respect for persons would then dictate that prisoners be protected. Whether to allow prisoners to "volunteer" or to "protect" them presents a dilemma. Respecting persons, in most hard cases, is often a matter of balancing competing claims urged by the principle of respect itself.

2. Beneficence. Persons are treated in an ethical manner not only by respecting their decisions and protecting them from harm, but also by making efforts to secure their well-being. Such treatment falls under the principle of beneficence. The term "beneficence" is often understood to cover acts of kindness or charity that go beyond strict obligation. In this document, beneficence is understood in a stronger sense, as an obligation. Two general rules have been formulated as complementary expressions of beneficent actions in this sense: **(1)** do not harm and **(2)** maximize possible benefits and minimize possible harms.

The Hippocratic maxim "do no harm" has long been a fundamental principle of medical ethics. Claude Bernard extended it to the realm of research, saying that one should not injure one person regardless of the benefits that might come to others. However, even avoiding harm requires learning what is harmful; and, in the process of obtaining this information, persons may be exposed to risk of harm. Further, the Hippocratic Oath requires physicians to benefit their patients "according to their best judgment." Learning what will in fact benefit may require exposing persons to risk. The problem posed by these imperatives is to decide when it is justifiable to seek certain benefits despite the risks involved, and when the benefits should be foregone because of the risks.

The obligations of beneficence affect both individual investigators and society at large, because they extend both to particular research projects and to the entire enterprise of research. In the case of particular projects, investigators and members of their institutions are obliged to give forethought to the maximization of benefits and the reduction of risk that might occur from the research investigation. In the case of scientific research in general, members of the larger society are obliged to recognize the longer term benefits and risks that may result from the improvement of knowledge and from the development of novel medical, psychotherapeutic, and social procedures.

The principle of beneficence often occupies a well-defined justifying role in many areas of research involving human subjects. An example is found in research involving children. Effective ways of treating childhood diseases and fostering healthy development are benefits that serve to justify research involving children—even when individual research subjects are not direct beneficiaries. Research also makes it possible to avoid the harm that may result from the application of previously accepted routine practices that on closer investigation turn out to be dangerous. But the role of the principle of beneficence is not always so unambiguous. A difficult ethical problem remains, for example, about research that presents more than minimal risk without immediate prospect of direct benefit to the children involved. Some have argued that such research is inadmissible, while others have pointed out that this limit would rule out much research promising great benefit to children in the future. Here again, as with all hard cases, the different claims covered by the principle of beneficence may come into conflict and force difficult choices.

Table 7-3 (Continued)

3. Justice. Who ought to receive the benefits of research and bear its burdens? This is a question of justice, in the sense of "fairness in distribution" or "what is deserved." An injustice occurs when some benefit to which a person is entitled is denied without good reason or when some burden is imposed unduly. Another way of conceiving the principle of justice is that equals ought to be treated equally. However, this statement requires explication. Who is equal and who is unequal? What considerations justify departure from equal distribution? Almost all commentators allow that distinctions based on experience, age, deprivation, competence, merit and position do sometimes constitute criteria justifying differential treatment for certain purposes. It is necessary, then, to explain in what respects people should be treated equally. There are several widely accepted formulations of just ways to distribute burdens and benefits. Each formulation mentions some relevant property on the basis of which burdens and benefits should be distributed. These formulations are **(1)** to each person an equal share, **(2)** to each person according to individual need, **(3)** to each person according to individual effort, **(4)** to each person according to societal contribution, and **(5)** to each person according to merit.

Questions of justice have long been associated with social practices such as punishment, taxation and political representation. Until recently these questions have not generally been associated with scientific research. However, they are foreshadowed even in the earliest reflections on the ethics of research involving human subjects. For example, during the 19th and early 20th centuries the burdens of serving as research subjects fell largely upon poor ward patients, while the benefits of improved medical care flowed primarily to private patients. Subsequently, the exploitation of unwilling prisoners as research subjects in Nazi concentration camps was condemned as a particularly flagrant injustice. In this country, in the 1940's, the Tuskegee syphilis study used disadvantaged, rural black men to study the untreated course of a disease that is by no means confined to that population. These subjects were deprived of demonstrably effective treatment in order not to interrupt the project, long after such treatment became generally available.

Against this historical background, it can be seen how conceptions of justice are relevant to research involving human subjects. For example, the selection of research subjects needs to be scrutinized in order to determine whether some classes (eg, welfare patients, particular racial and ethnic minorities, or persons confined to institutions) are being systematically selected simply because of their easy availability, their compromised position, or their manipulability, rather than for reasons directly related to the problem being studied. Finally, whenever research supported by public funds leads to the development of therapeutic devices and procedures, justice demands both that these not provide advantages only to those who can afford them and that such research should not unduly involve persons from groups unlikely to be among the beneficiaries of subsequent applications of the research.

Part C: Applications

C. Applications

Applications of the general principles to the conduct of research leads to consideration of the following requirements: informed consent, risk/benefit assessment, and the selection of subjects of research.

Table 7-3 (Continued)

1. Informed Consent. Respect for persons requires that subjects, to the degree that they are capable, be given the opportunity to choose what shall or shall not happen to them. This opportunity is provided when adequate standards for informed consent are satisfied.

While the importance of informed consent is unquestioned, controversy prevails over the nature and possibility of an informed consent. Nonetheless, there is widespread agreement that the consent process can be analyzed as containing three elements: information, comprehension and voluntariness.

Information. Most codes of research establish specific items for disclosure intended to assure that subjects are given sufficient information. These items generally include: the research procedure, their purposes, risks and anticipated benefits, alternative procedures (where therapy is involved), and a statement offering the subject the opportunity to ask questions and to withdraw at any time from the research. Additional items have been proposed, including how subjects are selected, the person responsible for the research, etc.

However, a simple listing of items does not answer the question of what the standard should be for judging how much and what sort of information should be provided. One standard frequently invoked in medical practice, namely the information commonly provided by practitioners in the field or in the locale, is inadequate since research takes place precisely when a common understanding does not exist. Another standard, currently popular in malpractice law, requires the practitioner to reveal the information that reasonable persons would wish to know in order to make a decision regarding their care. This, too, seems insufficient since the research subject, being in essence a volunteer, may wish to know considerably more about risks gratuitously undertaken than do patients who deliver themselves into the hand of a clinician for needed care. It may be that a standard of "the reasonable volunteer" should be proposed: the extent and nature of information should be such that persons, knowing that the procedure is neither necessary for their care nor perhaps fully understood, can decide whether they wish to participate in the furthering of knowledge. Even when some direct benefit to them is anticipated, the subjects should understand clearly the range of risk and the voluntary nature of participation.

A special problem of consent arises where informing subjects of some pertinent aspect of the research is likely to impair the validity of the research. In many cases, it is sufficient to indicate to subjects that they are being invited to participate in research of which some features will not be revealed until the research is concluded. In all cases of research involving incomplete disclosure, such research is justified only if it is clear that **(1)** incomplete disclosure is truly necessary to accomplish the goals of the research, **(2)** there are no undisclosed risks to subjects that are more than minimal, and **(3)** there is an adequate plan for debriefing subjects, when appropriate, and for dissemination of research results to them. Information about risks should never be withheld for the purpose of eliciting the cooperation of subjects, and truthful answers should always be given to direct questions about the research. Care should be taken to distinguish cases in which disclosure would destroy or invalidate the research from cases in which disclosure would simply inconvenience the investigator.

Table 7-3 (Continued)

Comprehension. The manner and context in which information is conveyed is as important as the information itself. For example, presenting information in a disorganized and rapid fashion, allowing too little time for consideration or curtailing opportunities for questioning, all may adversely affect a subject's ability to make an informed choice.

Because the subject's ability to understand is a function of intelligence, rationality, maturity and language, it is necessary to adapt the presentation of the information to the subject's capacities. Investigators are responsible for ascertaining that the subject has comprehended the information. While there is always an obligation to ascertain that the information about risk to subjects is complete and adequately comprehended, when the risks are more serious, that obligation increases. On occasion, it may be suitable to give some oral or written tests of comprehension.

Special provision may need to be made when comprehension is severely limited—for example, by conditions of immaturity or mental disability. Each class of subjects that one might consider as incompetent (eg, infants and young children, mentally disable patients, the terminally ill and the comatose) should be considered on its own terms. Even for these persons, however, respect requires giving them the opportunity to choose to the extent they are able, whether or not to participate in research. The objections of these subjects to involvement should be honored, unless the research entails providing them a therapy unavailable elsewhere. Respect for persons also requires seeking the permission of other parties in order to protect the subjects from harm. Such persons are thus respected both by acknowledging their own wishes and by the use of third parties to protect them from harm.

The third parties chosen should be those who are most likely to understand the incompetent subject's situation and to act in that person's best interest. The person authorized to act on behalf of the subject should be given an opportunity to observe the research as it proceeds in order to be able to withdraw the subject from the research, if such action appears in the subject's best interest.

Voluntariness. An agreement to participate in research constitutes a valid consent only if voluntarily given. This element of informed consent requires conditions free of coercion and undue influence. Coercion occurs when an overt threat of harm is intentionally presented by one person to another in order to obtain compliance. Undue influence, by contrast, occurs through an offer of an excessive, unwarranted, inappropriate or improper reward or other overture in order to obtain compliance. Also, inducements that would ordinarily be acceptable may become undue influences if the subject is especially vulnerable.

Unjustifiable pressures usually occur when persons in positions of authority or commanding influence—especially where possible sanctions are involved—urge a course of action for a subject. A continuum of such influencing factors exists, however, and it is impossible to state precisely where justifiable persuasion ends and undue influence begins. But undue influence would include actions such as manipulating a person's choice through the controlling influence of a close relative and threatening to withdraw health services to which an individual would otherwise be entitled.

2. Assessment of Risks and Benefits. The assessment of risks and benefits requires a careful array of relevant data, including, in some cases, alternative ways of obtaining the

Table 7-3 (Continued)

benefits sought in the research. Thus, the assessment presents both an opportunity and a responsibility to gather systematic and comprehensive information about proposed research. For the investigator, it is a means to examine whether the proposed research is properly designed. For a review committee, it is a method for determining whether the risks that will be presented to subjects are justified. For prospective subjects, the assessment will assist the determination whether or not to participate.

The Nature and Scope of Risks and Benefits. The requirement that research be justified on the basis of a favorable risk/benefit assessment bears a close relation to the principle of beneficence, just as the moral requirement that informed consent be obtained is derived primarily from the principle of respect for persons. The term "risk" refers to a possibility that harm may occur. However, when expressions such as "small risk" or "high risk" are used, they usually refer (often ambiguously) both to the chance (probability) of experiencing a harm and the severity (magnitude) of the envisioned harm.

The term "benefit" is used in the research context to refer to something of positive value related to health or welfare. Unlike "risk," "benefit" is not a term that expresses probabilities. Risk is properly contrasted to probability of benefits, and benefits are properly contrasted with harms rather than risks of harm. Accordingly, so-called risk/benefit assessments are concerned with the probabilities and magnitudes of possible harm and anticipated benefits. Many kinds of possible harms and benefits need to be taken into account. There are, for example, risks of psychological harm, physical harm, legal harm, social harm and economic harm and the corresponding benefits. While the most likely types of harms to research subjects are those of psychological or physical pain or injury, other possible kinds should not be overlooked.

Risks and benefits of research may affect the individual subjects, the families of the individual subjects, and society at large (or special groups of subjects in society). Previous codes and Federal regulations have required that risks to subjects be outweighed by the sum of both the anticipated benefit to the subject, if any, and the anticipated benefit to society in the form of knowledge to be gained from the research. In balancing these different elements, the risks and benefits affecting the immediate research subject will normally carry special weight. On the other hand, interests other than those of the subject may on some occasions be sufficient by themselves to justify the risks involved in the research, so long as the subjects' rights have been protected. Beneficence thus requires that we protect against risk of harm to subjects and also that we be concerned about the loss of the substantial benefits that might be gained from research.

The Systematic Assessment of Risks and Benefits. It is commonly said that benefits and risks must be "balanced" and shown to be "in a favorable ratio." The metaphorical character of these terms draws attention to the difficulty of making precise judgments. Only on rare occasions will quantitative techniques be available for the scrutiny of research protocols. However, the idea of systematic, nonarbitrary analysis of risks and benefits should be emulated insofar as possible. This ideal requires those making decisions about the justifiability of research to be thorough in the accumulation and assessment of information about all aspects of the research, and to consider alternatives systematically. This procedure renders the assessment of research more rigorous and precise, while making communication between review board members and investigators less subject to misinterpretation, misinformation and conflicting judgments. Thus, there

Table 7-3 (Continued)

should first be a determination of the validity of the presuppositions of the research; then the nature, probability and magnitude of risk should be distinguished with as much clarity as possible. The method of ascertaining risks should be explicit, especially where there is no alternative to the use of such vague categories as small or slight risk. It should also be determined whether an investigator's estimates of the probability of harm or benefits are reasonable, as judged by known facts or other available studies.

Finally, assessment of the justifiability of research should reflect at least the following considerations: **(i)** Brutal or inhumane treatment of human subjects is never morally justified. **(ii)** Risks should be reduced to those necessary to achieve the research objective. It should be determined whether it is in fact necessary to use human subjects at all. Risk can perhaps never be entirely eliminated, but it can often be reduced by careful attention to alternative procedures. **(iii)** When research involves significant risk of serious impairment, review committees should be extraordinarily insistent on the justification of the risk (looking usually to the likelihood of benefit to the subject—or, in some rare cases, to the manifest voluntariness of the participation). **(iv)** When vulnerable populations are involved in research, the appropriateness of involving them should itself be demonstrated. A number of variables go into such judgments, including the nature and degree of risk, the condition of the particular population involved, and the nature and level of the anticipated benefits. **(v)** Relevant risks and benefits must be thoroughly arrayed in documents and procedures used in the informed consent process.

3. Selection of Subjects. Just as the principle of respect for persons finds expression in the requirements for consent, and the principle of beneficence in risk/benefit assessment, the principle of justice gives rise to moral requirements that there be fair procedures and outcomes in the selection of research subjects.

Justice is relevant to the selection of subjects of research at two levels: the social and the individual. Individual justice in the selection of subjects would require that researchers exhibit fairness: thus, they should not offer potentially beneficial research only to some patients who are in their favor or select only "undesirable" persons for risky research. Social justice requires that distinction be drawn between classes of subjects that ought, and ought not, to participate in any particular kind of research, based on the ability of members of that class to bear burdens and on the appropriateness of placing further burdens on already burdened persons. Thus, it can be considered a matter of social justice that there is an order of preference in the selection of classes of subjects (eg, adults before children) and that some classes of potential subjects (eg, the institutionalized mentally infirm or prisoners) may be involved as research subjects, if at all, only on certain conditions.

Injustice may appear in the selection of subjects, even if individual subjects are selected fairly by investigators and treated fairly in the course of research. Thus injustice arises from social, racial, sexual and cultural biases institutionalized in society. Thus, even if individual researchers are treating their research subjects fairly, and even if IRBs are taking care to assure that subjects are selected fairly within a particular institution, unjust social patterns may nevertheless appear in the overall distribution of the burdens and benefits of research. Although individual institutions or investigators may not be able to resolve a problem that is pervasive in their social setting, they can consider distributive justice in selecting research subjects.

Table 7-3 (Continued)

Some populations, especially institutionalized ones, are already burdened in many ways by their infirmities and environments. When research is proposed that involves risks and does not include a therapeutic component, other less burdened classes of persons should be called upon first to accept these risks of research, except where the research is directly related to the specific conditions of the class involved. Also, even though public funds for research may often flow in the same directions as public funds for health care, it seems unfair that populations dependent on public health care constitute a pool of preferred research subjects if more advantaged populations are likely to be the recipients of the benefits.

One special instance of injustice results from the involvement of vulnerable subjects. Certain groups, such as racial minorities, the economically disadvantaged, the very sick, and the institutionalized may continually be sought as research subjects, owing to their ready availability in settings where research is conducted. Given their dependent status and their frequently compromised capacity for free consent, they should be protected against the danger of being involved in research solely for administrative convenience, or because they are easy to manipulate as a result of their illness or socioeconomic condition.

(A) Since 1945, various codes for the proper and responsible conduct of human experimentation in medical research have been adopted by different organizations. The best known of these codes are the Nuremberg Code of 1947, the Helsinki Declaration of 1964 (revised in 1975), and the 1971 Guidelines (codified into Federal Regulations in 1974) issued by the U.S. Department of Health, Education, and Welfare. Codes for the conduct of social and behavioral research have also been adopted, the best known being that of the American Psychological Association, published in 1973.

(B) Although practice usually involves interventions designed solely to enhance the well-being of a particular individual, interventions are sometimes applied to one individual for the enhancement of the well-being of another (eg, blood donation, skin grafts, organ transplants) or an intervention may have the dual purpose of enhancing the well-being of a particular individual, and, at the same time, providing some benefit to others (eg, vaccination, which protects both the person who is vaccinated and society generally). The fact that some forms of practice have elements other than immediate benefit to the individual receiving an intervention, however, should not confuse the general distinction between research and practice. Even when a procedure applied in practice may benefit some other person, it remains an intervention designed to enhance the well-being of a particular individual or groups of individuals; thus, it is practice and need not be reviewed as research.

(C) Because the problems related to social experimentation may differ substantially from those of biomedical and behavioral research, the Commission specifically declines to make any policy determination regarding such research at this time. Rather, the Commission believes that the problem ought to be addressed by one of its successor bodies.

REFERENCES

1. *Trials of War Criminals before the Nuremberg Military Tribunals under Control Council Law No. 10.* Vol 2. Washington, DC: US Government Printing Office; 1949:181-182.

2. World Medical Association recommendations guiding physicians in biomedical research involving human subjects. Available at: http://www.wma.net/e/17-c_eprargraphnumbering.html. Accessed July 18, 2000.

3. The Belmont Report: Ethical Principles and Guidelines for the Protection of Human Subjects of Research. Available at: http://www.grants.nih.gov/grants/oprr/humansubjects/guidance/belmont.htm. Accessed July 18, 2000.

4. Federal Policy for the Protection of Human Rights (45 CFR 46). Available at: http://www.grants.nih.gov/grants/oprr/humansubjects/45cfr46.htm. Accessed July 18, 2000.

5. The Institutional Review Board Guidebook (IRB Guidebook, revised 1993). Available at: http://ohrp.osophs.dhhs.gov/irb/irb_guidebook.htm. Accessed July 18, 2000.

RECOMMENDED READING

Appelbaum PS, Rosenbaum A. Tarasoff and the researcher: does the duty to protect apply in the research setting? *Am Psychol.* 1989;44(6):885-894.

Appelbaum PS, Roth LH, Detre T, et al. Researchers' access to patient records: an analysis of the ethical problems. *Clinical Research.* 1984;32(4):399-403.

Baumrind D. Research using intentional deception: ethical issues revisited. *Am Psychol.* 1985;40(2):165-174.

Beauchamp TL. Ethical theory and epidemiology. *J Clin Epidemiol.* 1991;44(supplI):S5-S8.

Beauchamp TL, Cook RR, Fayerweather WE, et al. Appendix: ethical guidelines for epidemiologists. *J Clin Epidemiol.* 1991;44(supplI):S151-S169.

Beecher HK. Ethics and clinical research. *N Engl J Med.* 1966;274:1354-1360.

Bordas LM. Tort liability of institutional review boards. *West Virginia Law Review.* 1984;87(1):137-164.

Brazzell RK, Colburn WA. Controversy I: patients or healthy volunteers for pharmacokinetic studies? *J Clin Pharmacol.* 1986;26(4):242-254.

Brett A, Grodin M. Ethical aspects of human experimentation in health services research. *JAMA.* 1991;265(14):1854-1857.

Brock DW, Wartman SA. When competent patients make irrational choices. *N Engl J Med.* 1990;322(22):1595-1599.

Buck BA. Ethical issues of randomized clinical trials. *Radiol Technol.* 1990;61(3):202-205.

Cassileth BR, Zupkis RV, Sutton-Smith K, March V. Informed consent—why are its goals imperfectly realized? *N Engl J Med.* 1980;302(16):896-900.

Chalmers TC. Ethical implications of rejecting patients for clinical trials. *JAMA.* 1990;263(6):865.

Culliton BJ. Human experimentation: AIDS trials questioned. *Nature.* 1991;350(6316):263.

Delgado R, Leskovac H. Informed consent in human experimentation: bridging the gap between ethical thought and current practice. *UCLA Law Review.* 1986;34(1):67-130.

Ellenberg SS. Randomization designs in comparative clinical trials. *N Engl J Med.* 1984;310(21):1404-1408.

Euretig JG. Legal and ethical aspects of deliberate G-induced loss of consciousness experiments. *Aviat Space Environ Med.* 1991;62(7):628-631.

Freedman B. Equipoise and the ethics of clinical research. *N Engl J Med.* 1987;317(3):141-145.

Giammona M, Glantz SA. Poor statistical design in research on humans: the role of committees in human research. *Clinical Research.* 1983;31(5):572-578.

Gifford F. The conflict between randomized clinical trials and the therapeutic obligation. *J Med Philos.* 1986;11(4):347-366.

Gordis L, Gold E. Privacy, confidentiality, and the use of medical records in research. *Science.* 1980;207(Jan 11):153-156.

Gostin L. Ethical principles for the conduct of human subject research: population-based research and ethics. *Law, Medicine and Health Care.* 1991;19(3-4):191-201.

Grodin MA, Zaharoff BE, Kaminow PV. A 12-year audit of IRB decisions. *QRB/Quality Review Bulletin.* 1986;12(3):82-86.

Johnson N, Lilford RJ, Brazier W. At what level of collective equipoise does a clinical trial become ethical? *J Med Ethics.* 1991;17(1):30-34.

Kadane JB. Progress toward a more ethical method for clinical trials. *J Med Philos.* 1986;11(4):385-404.

Kravitz R. Serving several masters: conflicting responsibilities in health services research. *J Gen Intern Med.* 1990;5(2):170-174.

Levine RJ. Apparent incompatibility between informed consent and placebo-controlled clinical trials. *Clin Pharmacol Ther.* 1987;42(3):247-49.

Levine RJ. Informed consent in research and practice: similarities and differences. *Arch Intern Med.* 1983;143(5):1229-1231.

Lind SE. Can patients be asked to pay for experimental treatment? *Clinical Research.* 1984;32(4):393-398.

Llewellyn-Thomas HA, Thiel EC, Clark RM. Patients versus surrogates: whose opinion counts on ethics review panels? *Clinical Research.* 1989;37(3):501-505.

Mackillop WJ, Johnston PA. Ethical problems in clinical research: the need for empirical studies of the clinical trials process. *Journal of Chronic Diseases.* 1986;39(3):177-188.

Melton GB. Ethical and legal issues in research and intervention. *J Adoles Health.* 1989;10(suppl3):S36-S44.

Newell JD. The case for deception in medical experimentation. *Philosophy in Context.* 1984;14:51-59.

Rosner F. Risk-benefit ratio: hazardous surgery and experimental therapy. *Mt Sinai J Med.* 1984;51(1):58-59.

Rosser SV. Re-visioning clinical research: gender and the ethics of experimental design. *Hypatia.* 1989;4(2):125-139.

Schwartz RL. Institutional review of medical research: cost-benefit analysis, risk-benefit analysis, and the possible effects of research on public policy. *J Leg Med.* 1983;4(2):143-166.

Spivey WH. Informed consent for clinical research in the emergency department. *Ann Emerg Med.* 1989;18(7):766-771.

Veatch RM. The patient as partner: ethics in clinical oncology research. *The Johns Hopkins Medical Journal.* 1982;151(4):155-161.

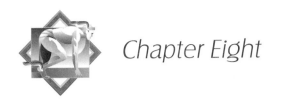

Chapter Eight

Publishing Athletic Training Research

"If you can't explain it simply, you don't understand it well enough." —Albert Einstein

Many describe how to publish research, but few explain why it is important; perhaps thinking it is self-evident. I am unwilling to take the risk of omitting this point, so here is my attempt at expounding the importance of publishing research.

Imagine that you have developed the most effective treatment that the world has ever seen for an athletic injury but never shared it with anyone. Every time you use the treatment, you get perfect results. You see this type of injury about 50 times per year (awfully high incidence rate, but bear with me). You enjoy your career in athletic training for 30 years after your discovery of this treatment. Fifteen hundred athletes benefit from your treatment in your lifetime. Given that this injury occurs 250,000 times per year nationwide, 7,500,000 people could have benefited in the 30 years since you discovered this treatment. Put another way, 7,498,500 athletes did not benefit from your treatment because you did not share it! Most responsible clinicians do share their techniques with coworkers, so the actual number would not be this high, but it would still be much lower than if you published your results. If you had published your treatment plan and 200 people read it and they had 30 more years of service, 300,000 athletes could have benefited.

People rarely find a perfect treatment plan; however, sharing your findings is still important. Your ideas may serve as a springboard for other more effective treatment plans. If these ideas are never published, they will serve a relatively small percentage of those who could have benefited if the idea had been shared. So, in a larger sense, ideas that are not shared are not helpful because no one can benefit from them.

There are basically five types of papers published in the athletic training literature: original research, literature reviews, case reports, clinical techniques, and communications. Original research papers, or experimental reports, are presentations of research performed by the authors. In a literature review, authors review other papers and draw conclusions about the current state of the literature in a certain area. Case reports are presentations of cases that are unique in some way; either the injury/condition is unique or the way it is handled is unique. Clinical techniques present specific techniques that authors have developed and are usually supported with current literature. Communications are opinion papers.

Each type of paper is presented differently to represent its content. There are two issues to discuss in regard to preparing manuscripts for publication: structure and presentation. The structure has to do with what goes where. Presentation has to do with clearly communicating your ideas.

STRUCTURE OF A MANUSCRIPT

Although each type of manuscript is unique, all share the following elements: title page, acknowledgments, abstract, text, references, tables, and illustrations. It is important to read the "Author's

Guide" for the journal to which you submit your manuscript, as well as the style manual the journal uses, which determines the specific structure required.

Title Page

Titles should be brief and concise, include the name of the disability or treatment technique if applicable, and reflect the outcome of the study.[1] Phrases like "The effects of," "A comparison of," "The treatment of," and "Reports of a case of" should not be used.[2] Title pages generally include the names, credentials, affiliations, and contact information of the authors.

Acknowledgments

This section is designed to thank those who helped with the study but are not included as authors. You may identify someone who made suggestions to your manuscript, identify a funding source, etc.

Abstract

Most journals require a comprehensive abstract regardless of the type of paper submitted. These abstracts are typically 75 to 300 words. Most sports medicine journals now require structured abstracts. Abstracts are structured differently depending on the type of manuscript. Abstract structuring recommended in the *AMA Manual of Style*[2] is as follows: Original research papers—Context, Objective, Design, Setting, Patients or Other Participants, Intervention(s), Main Outcome Measure(s), Results, Conclusions; Literature review—Objective, Data Sources, Study Selection, Data Extraction, Data Synthesis, and Conclusions. Knight and Ingersoll[1] recommend structured abstract headings for case reports (Objective, Background, Differential Diagnosis, Treatment, Uniqueness, and Conclusions) and clinical techniques (Objective, Background, Description, and Clinical Advantages). Some journals also require a listing of key terms.

Text

The text, or body, of a manuscript depends on the type of manuscript. The article's relevant information is presented in the text. This is the "guts" of the paper.

ORIGINAL RESEARCH PAPERS

The text for an original research paper typically follows the acronym IMRAD (Introduction, Methods, Results, and Discussion). The *introduction* develops the problem to be studied, stimulates interest in the subject, develops both sides of a controversy, and culminates in a specific statement of the purpose of the study. The introduction section should be brief and to the point. Provide enough information to develop the controversy but not so much that a reader would lose interest.

The *methods* section is often broken up into four or five subsections. They include an introductory paragraph describing the study's design, subjects, instruments, testing procedures, and statistical analysis. The introductory paragraph provides a roadmap for the study. The factorial, the independent variable(s), and its levels, the dependent variable(s), are specifically identified. This helps the reader understand the overall set-up of the study before delving further into the methods section.

The *subjects* subsection describes the subjects, human, animal, or otherwise, used in the study. Demographic information such as age, height, weight, activity level, gender, etc, is presented. Information regarding inclusion or exclusion criteria, securing of informed consent, and approval from an IRB for use of human subjects in the research is also presented. When using human subjects, a clarification stating subjects are volunteers is usually included as well.

The *instruments* subsection is used to describe the instruments used in the study. It is not to describe how the instruments were used, which goes in the procedures subsection, but does describe the model number, manufacturer, and general measurement capabilities of the instruments. The idea is to give the reader enough information about your instruments so that they can find the same or similar instruments for their studies if they so wish.

The *testing procedures* subsection describes how the study was conducted. Step-by-step descriptions, bulleted points if possible, help the reader understand what you did in the study. It should be detailed enough that someone could repeat your experiment by reading your testing procedures. Photographs or line drawings are sometimes helpful to convey testing setups.

The *statistical analysis* subsection identifies the specific statistical tests used to analyze the research data. These often include main analyses and post hoc tests. Identifying the probability level you are accepting is often included.

The *results* section is used to present the outcome of your study. The results section is not the place where you try to explain why the study turned out the way it did. Rather, you simply describe what happened. Descriptive statistics are often presented first. Organizing the rest of the results section based on the outcome of statistical tests often provides a logical sequencing. Copious use of tables and figures is recommended, as it helps convey the meaning of the data; however, text and tables or figures should not be redundant.

In the *discussion* section you interpret your findings, fit them in to what is already known, and make conclusions. Interpreting your findings means that you explain the results. Fitting your results into what is already known means that you describe how your findings fit into current theory and compare your findings to what others have done. In making conclusions, specifically state what you think your results mean and recommend or suggest applications of your findings. Be sure to discuss your results and not what you wished or thought they would be.

LITERATURE REVIEW PAPERS

Literature review papers generally include an introduction, a body, and a conclusion. The introduction serves much the same purpose it did for original research papers. It stimulates interest and specifically identifies the area(s) you are going to review. The body includes subheadings containing reviews of relevant information. More general information is presented toward the beginning and more specific or specialized information is presented toward the end. Emphasize the information you are presenting, not the authors you are citing. Critically review the literature. Do not simply restate what other authors said. Do not be afraid to criticize a study that you feel is flawed, but be sure to clearly identify why you think it is flawed. When drawing conclusions, be clear and concise, and make sure your conclusions are based on the literature you reviewed.

CASE STUDY

The body of a case study should include personal data, chief complaint, history of present complaint, results of physical examination, medical history, diagnosis, treatment, clinical course, criteria for return to competition, and deviation from the expected.

CLINICAL TECHNIQUE

A clinical technique should include the how and why of the technique. Step-by-step explanations of how to perform the technique should be supported by the literature when possible and supplemented by photographs and illustrations. Similar techniques should be reviewed, and the advantages and disadvantages of your technique should be compared to others.

References/Citations

References are journal articles, textbooks, abstracts, etc, from the literature. A reference is presented as a bibliographic entry. All references are listed in a *references* section following the body of the manuscript. References are organized differently depending on the type (ie, journal article, book, dissertation, etc) and the referencing style (eg, AMA, American Psychological Association [APA]). Examples of different types of references in AMA style follow. Number 1 is a journal article, 2 is a book, 3 is a book chapter, and 4 is a presentation. Referencing for this book uses AMA format.

1. Knight KL, Ingersoll CD. Optimizing scholarly communication: 30 tips for writing clearly. *J Athl Train.* 1996;31:209-213.

2. Day DA. *Scientific English: A Guide for Scientists and Other Professionals.* 2nd ed. Phoenix, Ariz: Oryx Press; 1995:73-74.

3. Leadbetter WB. An introduction to sports-induced soft-tissue inflammation. In: Leadbetter WB, Buckwalter JA, Gordon SL, eds. *Sports-Induced Inflammation.* Park Ridge, Ill: American Academy of Orthopaedic Surgeons; 1990:3-23.

4. Stone JA. Swiss ball rehabilitation exercises. Presented at the 47th Annual Meeting and Clinical Symposium of the National Athletic Trainers' Association; June 12, 1996; Orlando, Fla.

References are typically listed either alphabetically or in the order of citation, again depending on the style manual followed.

Citations are mentions of references in the paper. These mentions are denoted in the text either by the author(s)'s name(s) and year of publication, as in APA style, or using reference numbers, as in AMA or Council of Biology Editors (CBE) style. It is important to read the style manual or authors' guide of the journal to correctly cite references.

Citations should be used liberally. It is important to give appropriate credit for others' ideas because failure to do so is plagiarism. To plagiarize is to steal and use the ideas or writings of another as one's own.[3] Don't plagiarize!

Tables and Illustrations

The purpose of tables is to centralize large amounts of data, save space, and eliminate long paragraphs of forced and redundant text.[1] Tables should:
*   Be understandable without referring to the text
*   Identify units of measurement in the most general way possible (usually in parentheses in column headers)
*   Include measures of central tendency (means, medians, modes) and variability (standard deviations, standard errors)

Tables should not:
*   Be redundant with the text
*   Include information that can be easily included within the text (eg, subject information)
*   Contain vertical lines

Illustrations are often helpful in presenting concepts that are difficult to describe, such as testing set-ups, x-ray abnormalities, and even trends within data. Illustrations may be photographs, line drawings, flow charts, charts, graphs, or the like. Clear and descriptive legends should be provided to describe what is contained in the illustration and/or to point out salient points that you want the reader to notice.

A legend of tables and illustrations (sometimes called figures) is generally included at the end of a manuscript.

For More Help

I recommend reading *How to Write & Publish a Scientific Paper,*[4] the *AMA Manual of Style,*[1] *Scientific Style and Format: The CBE Manual for Authors, Editors, and Publishers,*[5] and the authors' guides in the journal to which you are submitting a manuscript. Table 8-1 contains world wide web addresses for sports medicine journals. Authors' Guides for many of these journals are included on their web pages.

Table 8-1

Some Journals Relevant to Athletic Training Research

Journal Name	ISSN	Publisher	Publication Frequency	Web Address
American Journal of Physical Medicine & Rehabilitation	0894-9115	Lippincott Williams & Wilkins	Bimonthly	www.physiatry.org/publications/
American Journal of Sports Medicine	0363-5465	Williams & Wilkins	Bimonthly	www.sportsmed.org/journal/default.htm
Archives of Physical Medicine and Rehabilitation	0003-9993	WB Saunders Company	Monthly	www.archives-pmr.org/
Athletic Therapy Today	1078-7895	Human Kinetics Publishers, Inc.	Bimonthly	www.hkusa.com/
British Journal of Sports Medicine	0306-3674	BMJ Publishing Group	Bimonthly	www.bjsportmed.com/
Clinical Biomechanics	0268-0033	Elsevier Science	10 issues/year	www.elsevier.nl/
Clinical Journal of Sports Medicine	1050-642X	Lippincott Williams & Wilkins	Quarterly	www.cjsportmed.com
Gait & Posture	0966-6362	Elsevier Science	Bimonthly	www.elsevier.nl/
International Journal of Sports Medicine	0172-4622	Thieme Journals	8 issues/year	www.thieme.com/onGJJMAFIKHLKI/display/762
Isokinetics and Exercise Science	0959-3020	Elsevier Science	Quarterly	N/A
Journal of Athletic Training	1062-6050	National Athletic Trainers' Association	Quarterly	www.journalofathletictraining.org/

Table 8-1 (Continued)

Journal Name	ISSN	Publisher	Publication Frequency	Web Address
Journal of Electromyography and Kinesiology	1050-6411	Elsevier Science	Bimonthly	www.elsevier.nl/
Journal of Orthopaedic and Sports Physical Therapy	0190-6011	Orthopaedic and Sports Physical Therapy Sections of the APTA	Monthly	N/A
Journal of Sport Rehabilitation	1056-6716	Human Kinetics Publishers, Inc.	Quarterly	www.hkusa.com/
Journal of Sports Medicine and Physical Fitness	0022-4707	Minerva Medica	Quarterly	www.minervamedica.it/goingl2_ita.html
Medicine and Science in Sports and Exercise	0195-9131	Lippincott Williams & Wilkins	Monthly	www.ms-se.com/
The Physician and Sportsmedicine	0091-3847	McGraw-Hill Companies	Monthly	www.physsportsmed.com/
Sports Medicine	0112-1642	Adis International	Monthly	www.adis.com/
Sports Medicine and Arthroscopy Review	1062-8592	Lippincott Williams & Wilkins	Quarterly	www.sportsmedarthro.com/
Sports Medicine, Training and Rehabilitation	1057-8315	Harwood Academic Publishers	Quarterly	www.gbhap.com/journals/353/353-top.htm/

Table 8-2	
EXAMPLES OF ACTIVE AND PASSIVE VOICE	
Active Voice	Passive Voice
Priscilla *applied* the brace.	The brace *was applied* by Priscilla.
We *measured* the temperature every 5 minutes.	The temperature *was measured* every 5 minutes by the authors of the study.

WRITING WITH STYLE

The best idea in the world is useless unless it can be communicated clearly. Clear communication must be the prime objective of scientific writing.[6] Content, structure, and clarity of presentation are the major elements of effective scholarly communication.[7] Content comes from what you know about the subject. Structure was discussed in the previous section. Clarity of presentation is presented here.

Grammar

Voice, person, tense, number, and parallelism are five critical elements of grammar that are important in scientific writing. Voice refers to the action of a verb, which can be active or passive. A verb with a direct object is in the active voice. When the direct object is converted into a subject, the verb is in the passive voice. A passive verb is always a verb phrase consisting of a form of the verb *be* (usually was) followed by a past participle. The subject of a passive verb does not act. In each of the examples in Table 8-2, my word processor noted that sentences in the passive voice were grammatically incorrect. The suggested correction was similar to the active voice example.

The active voice is preferred in scientific writing.[7-10] The passive voice is dry, dull, rigid, pompous, ambiguous,[8-11] weak, evasive, convoluting, tentative, timid, sluggish, amateurish, obscene, and immoral.[12] The passive voice is often used to avoid using the personal pronoun "I," which is thought to be immodest. The passive voice does not sound more scientific or more objective. More often than not the passive voice introduces ambiguity, which is great if you do not want people to understand what you are saying.

Person is the form of a verb or a pronoun that indicates whether a person is speaking (first person), is spoken to (second person), or is spoken about (third person) (Table 8-3). Use first person when telling what you did, second person when describing how to perform a technique, and third person when explaining what others did.[7]

Tense relates a verb's relation in time. A verb's tense is represented by its inflection (eat, eats, eating, ate, eaten) and through the use of auxiliaries (will eat, have eaten, had eaten, will have eaten). Some general recommendations for using tense in a scientific manuscript are as follows:

- Use past tense when referring to events in the past
- Use present tense when giving instruction
- Use future tense when referring to events yet to occur

A common tense error is to represent others' work in something other than the past tense.

Parallelism describes when similar ideas are expressed in a similar, or parallel, fashion.[13] Nonparallelism often occurs in serial lists. The error is often an intermingling of noun phrases and verb phrases (see Table 8-4 for examples). One way to check for parallelism is to read the sentence including only one of the listed items at a time. If the truncated sentence does not make sense, it is probably not parallel.

Table 8-3

EXAMPLES OF FIRST, SECOND, AND THIRD PERSON

First Person

I see the boy.   *We* recommend this technique.

Second Person

Can *you* see the boy?   *(You* understood) Apply two strips vertically.

Third Person

He sees the boy.   *Each subject* lifted 100 lbs.

Table 8-4

EXAMPLES OF PARALLEL AND NONPARALLEL SENTENCES

Nonparallel	Parallel
The manufacturer claims the new dynamometer is more user-friendly *(a verb phrase)*, has more data storage capacity *(a verb phrase)*, and faster printing *(a noun phrase)*.	The manufacturer claims the new dynamometer is more user-friendly, has more storage capability, and prints faster.
Lachman's test is preferred over the anterior drawer test for evaluating anterior cruciate ligament tears because: 1. moving the knee to 90° is sometimes painful, 2. it negates the chance that joint mice will lock the joint, and 3. less influence of hamstring guarding.	Lachman's test is preferred over the anterior drawer test for evaluating anterior cruciate ligament tears because it: 1. is sometimes painful to move the knee to 90°, 2. negates the chance that joint mice will lock the joint, and 3. lessens the influence of hamstring guarding.

Writing Concisely

Vigorous writing is concise[14] and direct.[15] A sentence should contain no unnecessary words, and a paragraph should contain no unnecessary sentences.[14] This does not mean that all sentences and paragraphs should be short or lacking details but that every word should be purposeful.[14] Being as brief as possible, keeping vocabulary simple, avoiding abbreviations, and pruning empty words are all important in concise writing.

Here are some suggestions to help you write concisely[16]:

1. Present your points in logical order. Attempt to communicate your thoughts clearly with the fewest possible words.
2. Do not waste words telling people what they already know; however, be careful in your assumption of how much people know.
3. Cut out excess evidence and unnecessary anecdotes and examples.

Table 8-5

PRUNING WORDS

Poor	There are several techniques that could be utilized to tape an ankle.	It is my opinion that knee braces are helpful.
Better	The ankle can be taped several ways.	My opinion is that knee braces are useful.
Better still		I think knee braces are useful.

4. Look for windy phrases, which are the most common word wasters. For example, replace "at the present time" with "now" and "in the majority of instances" with "usually."
5. Look for passive verbs that you can make active. Invariably, this produces a shorter sentence.
6. When you've finished, stop.

Vocabulary should be kept simple. Day[17] condemned complicated vocabulary as follows:

1. "Thoughts are communicated more effectively with a forceful, simple, and direct vocabulary than with technical or scientific jargon and worship of polysyllables."[4]
2. "Long words name little things. All big things have little names, such as life and death, peace and war, or dawn, day, night, love, or home. Learn to use little words in a big way. It is hard to do, but they say what you mean. When you don't know what you mean, use big words. They often fool little people."[18]
3. "Big words can bog down; one may have to read them three or four times to make out what they mean. Short words are bright like sparks that glow in the night, moist like the sea that laps the shore, sharp like the blade of a knife, hot like salt tears that scald the cheek, quick like moths that flit from flame to flame, and terse like the dart and sting of a bee."[19]
4. "Too many scientists, and perhaps members of all professions, want to sound 'scholarly.' Therefore, they sometimes dress up a simple thought in an outrageous costume. Sometimes, the thread of the idea gets lost along the way, and all we see is the frayed costume. If I have learned anything from my years of experience in scientific writing, editing, and publishing, it is this: Simplicity of expression is a natural result of profound thought."[17]
5. "We have not known a single great scientist who could not discourse freely and interestingly with a child. Can it be that haters of clarity have nothing to say, have observed nothing, have no clear picture of even their own fields?"[20]

Most abbreviations, acronyms, and initialisms are strongly discouraged in scientific writing.[2,4,5,21,22] Only use abbreviations that are widely used and accepted.[2,4,5,22] SDULACAIYSW (so don't use long and confusing abbreviations in your scientific writing).

Prune all words that lack meaningful content.[16] Consider the pruning in Table 8-5.

Writing clearly is important in the published version of your thoughts. Do not let your attempts to write clearly interfere with your thinking. Allow yourself to have a draft that only you understand if it helps you get your ideas written down. Once you get your ideas down, then rework the manuscript so it is clearly written.

THESES AND DISSERTATIONS

Theses and dissertations should be prepared using the same general guidelines for style as presented above. The structure of theses and dissertations tends to be somewhat different from a journal manuscript, however. There are two general formats for theses and dissertations: the traditional or chapter format and the journal format.

The traditional or chapter format is generally organized as follows:

I. Front Matter
    A. Vita (often just for dissertations)
    B. Title page
    C. Approval sheet
    D. Abstract
    E. Acknowledgments
    F. Table of contents
    G. List of tables
    H. List of figures
II. Body
    A. Chapter 1: Introduction
        a. Statement of the problem
        b. Significance of the study
        c. Sources of data
        d. Limitations
        e. Assumptions
    B. Chapter 2: Review of Related Literature
        a. Description of sample
        b. Description of instruments used
        c. Data arrangement
        d. Data treatment
        e. Data analysis
    C. Chapter 3: Procedures
    D. Chapter 4: Results
    E. Chapter 5: Summary
        a. Conclusions
        b. Recommendations
III. Bibliography
IV. Appendix(es)
    A. Informed consent form
    B. Questionnaires
    C. Latin square tables
    D. Data collection sheets
    E. Specific testing procedures
    F. Other tables that augment information in Chapter 3: Procedures
    G. Table of raw data
    H. Statistical tables
    I. Other tables that augment information in Chapter 4: Results

The journal format is generally organized as follows:

I. Front Matter
    A. Vita (often just for dissertations)
    B. Title page
    C. Approval sheet
    D. Abstract
    E. Acknowledgments

F. Table of contents

G. List of tables

H. List of figures

II. Manuscript

    A. Introduction

    B. Methods

        a. Introductory paragraph

        b. Subjects

        c. Instruments

        d. Testing procedures

        e. Statistical analysis

    C. Results

    D. Discussion

    E. References

III. Appendices

    A. The problem

        a. Research question

        b. Experimental hypotheses

        c. Assumptions

        d. Delimitations

        e. Operational definitions

        f. Limitations

        g. Significance of the study

    B. Literature review

    C. Additional methods

        a. Informed consent form

        b. Questionnaires

        c. Latin square tables

        d. Data collection sheets

        e. Specific testing procedures

        f. Other tables that augment information in the Methods section of the manuscript

    D. Additional results

        a. Table of raw data

        b. Statistical tables

        c. Other tables that augment information in the Results section of the manuscript

    E. Recommendations for future research

IV. Bibliography (or Additional References)

    Bibliography references are cited only in the appendices and follow the references cited in the References section in the manuscript.

Which format should be used for your thesis or dissertation? To answer this question, you must first know what is available. Many academic departments prescribe the specific format for your thesis or dissertation, so you may have no choice. If that is the case, the following argument is moot. If you have a choice or you are in a position to recommend a format to your department, read on (you may want to read on anyway).

I will not try to hide my bias. I think the journal format is far superior to the traditional format for the following reasons:

    1. Theses and dissertations are supposed to prepare students to contribute to the knowledge base in their professions. With that in mind, why would you teach students to prepare a scientific manuscript in a format that is not typically used by journals (where research is published for most professions)?

2. Students learn to prepare journal manuscripts and will be better prepared to do so again in the future.

3. Students are familiar with manuscripts in journal format; therefore, they can concentrate on the research and not on how it has to be presented in their thesis/dissertation.

4. The journal format requires that students prepare all of the same materials as found in the traditional format so rigor is not lost in the process of making preparation easier.

5. Theses and dissertations prepared in the journal format are much easier to read; therefore people are more likely to read them.

6. Students do not have to do additional work to make their theses/dissertations ready to submit for publication. Students, particularly Masters-level students, are often too busy with their new jobs after finishing their theses or dissertations to invest a lot of time into changing a traditional format thesis around so it can be submitted for publication.

7. Because the journal format makes it easier for students to submit their theses or dissertations for publication, it decreases the likelihood that the thesis or dissertation advisor has to rework it him- or herself in order for it to be suitable for submission (okay, so this is a selfish reason).

At least one other author[23] agrees with me regarding thesis/dissertations formatting. The traditional method does have one advantage: it has a lot of tradition behind it (sorry, that is the best I could do).

SUBMITTING YOUR PAPER FOR PUBLICATION

Once you have finished writing your paper, you must then submit it for publication. The journal's author's guide will spell out how many copies are required, whether they should be paper or electronic, where to send the manuscripts, etc.

Once the editor receives your manuscript, he or she will either assign reviewers to evaluate the manuscript or assign an associate or section editor. The associate or section editor may then assign reviewers. The manuscript then goes to reviewers who evaluate it and make their recommendations to the editor. The editor then makes a decision regarding the suitability of the manuscript for publication. Publication recommendations are usually in one of four categories: publish as is, publish with minor modifications, make modifications and send back out for review, or reject. "Publish as is" occurs infrequently.

Generally, recommendations are made to modify your manuscript in some way. You must decide if you are willing to make the recommended changes and whether to resubmit. If you are unwilling to make the changes, you may consider sending the manuscript to another journal. If you are willing to make the changes and/or want to challenge the recommended changes, the manuscript should be resubmitted with a letter explaining how you addressed recommended changes. You then "haggle" with the editor until the manuscript is deemed appropriate for publication.

Occasionally, manuscripts are unconditionally rejected (meaning that the journal will not entertain another draft of that paper). This situation tests your confidence in your manuscript. Sometimes manuscripts are rejected because the topic is not considered appropriate for that journal or because the contents are considered flawed in some irreparable way. In either situation, you may consider submitting your paper to another journal (incorporating suggestions from the rejecting journal, of course).

Summary of Planning, Writing, and Publishing a Scientific Paper

Huth[21] succinctly described the process of preparing and publishing a manuscript in 20 steps:

1. Decide on the message of the paper. Can you state it in a single sentence? With case reports and reviews, you may not be sure of the exact message until you have searched the literature.
2. Decide whether the paper is worth writing. Have similar findings been reported? Is there a need for another report? With case reports and reviews, has your literature search turned up similar cases or reviews?
3. Decide on the importance of your paper. Apply the "so-what test"—how will the paper change a concept or a practice?
4. Decide on the audience for the paper; apply the "who-cares" test.
5. Select the journal for which you will prepare your paper.
6. Search the literature for a firm decision on writing the paper and its message and for documentary materials.
7. Decide on authorship and author order.
8. Assemble the materials needed to write and eventually publish the paper. If you are writing an invited review paper or editorial, make sure you know the conditions accompanying the invitation and request any you feel should be met before you accept.
9. Look up the manuscript requirements of the journal.
10. Consider the proper structure for the paper before you begin to outline it and write the first draft.
11. Develop a sketch or outline for the first draft.
12. Write the first draft.
13. Revise the draft and subsequent drafts (with any coauthors) until you are fully satisfied with the content of the paper.
14. Revise your prose for fluency, clarity, accuracy, economy, and grace.
15. Make sure that the details of scientific style are correct.
16. Prepare the final choices and correct presentations for tables and illustrations.
17. Review and revise, if necessary, the last complete draft and type the final manuscript.
18. Assemble the manuscript copies and accompanying materials to send to the journal's editor with a submission letter.
19. Respond to the editor's decision. Revise a provisionally accepted paper as requested, send a rejected paper to another journal after making needed revisions, or give up trying to get the paper published.
20. If the paper is accepted, correct the proof carefully as soon as it arrives, return it promptly, and await publication of the paper.

References

1. Knight KL, Ingersoll CD. Structure of a scholarly manuscript: 66 tips for what goes where. *J Athl Train*. 1996;31:201-206.
2. Iverson C, Flanagin A, Fontanarosa PB, et al. *American Medical Association Manual of Style*. 9th ed. Baltimore, Md: Williams & Wilkins; 1998.
3. Davies P, ed. *The American Heritage Dictionary of the English Language*. New York, NY: Dell Publishing Co; 1976:540.

4. Day RA. *How to Write & Publish a Scientific Paper.* 4th ed. Phoenix, Ariz: Oryx Press; 1994.

5. CBE Style Manual Committee. *CBE Style Manual: A Guide for Authors, Editors, and Publishers in the Biological Sciences.* 5th ed. Bethesda, Md: Council of Biology Editors, Inc; 1983:42.

6. Publication Manual of the American Psychological Association. Quoted by: Day RA. *Scientific English: A Guide for Scientists and Other Professionals.* 2nd ed. Phoenix, Ariz: Oryx Press; 1995:8.

7. Knight KL, Ingersoll CD. Optimizing scholarly communication: 30 tips for writing clearly. *J Athl Train.* 1996;31:209-213.

8. DeBakey L. Releasing literary inhibitions in scientific writing. *Can Med Assoc J.* 1968;99:360-367.

9. O'Connor M, Woodford FP. *Writing Scientific Papers in English.* New York, NY: Elsevier; 1976:21.

10. Tichy JH. *Effective Writing for Engineers, Managers, and Scientists.* New York, NY: John Wiley & Sons; 1966:197-198.

11. DeBakey L. Every careless word men utter. *Anesth Analg.* 1970;49:567-574.

12. Bush D. Quoted by: Day RA. *Scientific English: A Guide for Scientists and Other Professionals.* 2nd ed. Phoenix, Ariz: Oryx Press; 1995:72.

13. Fillmore ER, Hedegard K. Write it right. *ISN News.* 1988;9:28.

14. Strunk W, White EB. *The Elements of Style.* 3rd ed. New York, NY: Macmillan Publishing Co Inc; 1979:23.

15. Ebbitt WR, Ebbitt DR. Quoted by: Day RA. *Scientific English: A Guide for Scientists and Other Professionals.* 2nd ed. Phoenix, Ariz: Oryx Press; 1995:29.

16. Thompson ET. *How to Write Clearly.* Elmsford, NY: International Paper Company; 1979.

17. Day RA. *Scientific English: A Guide for Scientists and Other Professionals.* 2nd ed. Phoenix, Ariz: Oryx Press; 1995.

18. SSC Booknews. Quoted by: Day RA. *Scientific English: A Guide for Scientists and Other Professionals.* 2nd ed. Phoenix, Ariz: Oryx Press; 1995:21.

19. Wren C. Quoted by: Day RA. *Scientific English: A Guide for Scientists and Other Professionals.* 2nd ed. Phoenix, Ariz: Oryx Press; 1995:25.

20. Steinbeck J, Ricketts E. Quoted by: Day RA. *Scientific English: A Guide for Scientists and Other Professionals.* 2nd ed. Phoenix, Ariz: Oryx Press; 1995:8.

21. Huth EJ. *How to Write and Publish Papers in the Medical Sciences.* 2nd ed. Baltimore, Md: Williams & Wilkins; 1990:138.

22. Huth EJ. *Medical Style & Format.* Philadelphia, Pa: ISI Press; 1987:140-141.

23. Thomas JR, Nelson JK. *Research Methods in Physical Activity.* 3rd ed. Champaign, Ill: Human Kinetics; 1996:411-413.

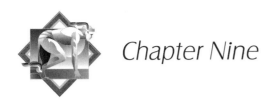

Chapter Nine

Fundamentals of Grant Writing

"I've always wanted to be a scientist. That way, I could get a bunch of grants and do research into whether money can really buy happiness." —Kyannke

Writing a grant proposal is a problem of persuasion. Assume that grant proposal readers are busy, impatient, skeptical people who have no reason to give your proposal special consideration and are faced with more requests than they can grant or even read thoroughly. Typically, grant proposal readers are looking for information that they can locate quickly and easily. Essentially, they are looking for the following[1]:

- What do you want to do, how much will it cost, and how much time will it take?
- How does the proposed project relate to the sponsor's interests?
- What difference will the project make to your university, your students, your discipline, the state, the nation, the world, or whatever appropriate categories? What has already been done in the area of your project?
- How do you plan to do it?
- How will the results be evaluated?
- Why should you, rather than someone else, do this project?

These questions are answered in different ways and receive different emphases depending on the nature of the proposed project and the agency to which the proposal is being submitted. Agencies generally provide detailed instructions or guidelines for proposal preparation. Some agencies actually provide forms on which the proposal must be typed, while others are moving toward electronic submissions. In any case, specific guidelines must be studied carefully before you begin writing the draft.

A successful grant application will convince reviewers that:

- Your proposed research will address important questions in an efficient and convincing way
- You know and understand pertinent literature in your field
- You have mastered all of the essential techniques needed to complete the stated research
- You have access to all of the equipment and supplies needed to complete the project
- You have budgeted appropriately to conduct and complete your project
- You will appropriately analyze and interpret the data
- You will complete your project in a timely fashion
- You will publish your work

FUNDING SOURCES

There are not many funding sources directly interested in funding athletic training research. There are more than most think, however. I was able to find information on six grant programs for athletic training research on the world wide web (Table 9-1). Check these websites before applying, as infor-

Table 9-1

FUNDING SOURCES FOR ATHLETIC TRAINING RESEARCH

Source	Annual Funds	Typical Award	Application Deadline(s)	Website Information
NATA Research & Education	Varies	$20,000 to $30,000*	September 1, March 1	www.natafoundation.org/
Eastern Athletic Trainers' Association	N/A	Up to $2000	April 1	www.goeata.org/
Great Lakes Athletic Trainers' Association	$3000	Up to $1000	February 1, June 1, October 1	www.glata.org/applications/ researchappl.html/
Far West Athletic Trainers' Association	$3000	$1000 to $1200	February 1	www.csuchico.edu/~sbarker/ FWATA/ricgrant.html/
Southeast Athletic Trainers' Association	$1500	Varies	February 15	www.seata.org/Grant/ grant.html/
Mid-America Athletic Trainers' Association	N/A	~$1000	January 15	N/A

This is for general grants program. Varies for request for proposals (RFPs) or other grant programs.

mation may change frequently. Further, eligibility for these grants is sometimes limited. For district association grants, you most likely will need to be a member of that district. Names of contact people may also be present. Do not be afraid to contact these people for additional information.

PARTS OF A PROPOSAL

Proposals for sponsored activities generally follow a similar format, although there are variations depending upon whether the author is seeking support for a research grant, a training grant, or a conference or curriculum development project.

Typical parts of a research proposal are:
1. Title page
2. Abstract
3. Table of contents
4. Introduction (including statement of problem, purpose of research, and significance of research)

5. Background (including literature survey)
6. Description of proposed research (including method or approach)
7. Description of relevant institutional resources
8. List of references
9. Personnel
10. Budget

Title Page

Most agencies specify the format for the title page and/or provide special forms to summarize basic administrative and fiscal data for the project. Title pages generally include signatures, typically from the principal investigator, his or her department head, and an official representing the university. The title page may also include the university's reference number for the proposal, the name of the agency to which the proposal is being submitted, the title of the proposal, the proposed starting date and budget period, the total funds requested, the name and address of the university unit submitting the proposal, and the date submitted. There may also be space to indicate whether the proposal is for a new or continuing project. You may also need to indicate whether this proposal has been submitted to other agencies.

A good title page also includes the title of the project. Titles should be comprehensive enough to indicate the nature of the proposed work, but they should also be brief. Cutting phrases like "Studies on...," "Investigations...," or "Research on Some Problems in...." helps shorten titles without compromising their meaning (see Chapter Eight for more writing tips).

Abstract

All proposals need abstracts. Many readers use the abstract as an overview of the project to remind them of its nature. Some readers rely very heavily on the abstract when making decisions on the whole proposal. As such, the abstract is very important. In fact, some agencies use the abstract in their compilations of research projects funded or in disseminating information about successful projects.

Though it appears first, the abstract should be written last. See Chapter Eight for more tips on writing an abstract.

To present the essential meaning of the proposal, the abstract should summarize the major objectives of the project and the procedures to be followed in meeting these objectives. The abstract must be able to be a stand-alone document. It is the single most important element in the proposal.

Table of Contents

A table of contents, a list of illustrations (or figures), and a list of tables may be required in more involved proposals. Refer to the agency's requirements for these elements.

Introduction

The introduction of a proposal should include a concise statement of what is being proposed and then should develop the problem. Do not assume that the reader will understand the nature of the problem you intend to study. You must convince him or her that it is an important problem. You must do this in a direct, easy-to-understand format.

Agency representatives may want to get a general idea of the proposed work before giving the proposal to reviewers who can judge its technical merit; thus, the introduction should be understandable to a reasonably informed layperson. The introduction should give enough background information to place your particular research problem in a context of common knowledge and should show how its solution will advance the field or be important for some other work. It is very important for you to state the importance of your research.

Background

A background section is not always needed. In cases where previous work must be discussed or pertinent literature must be reviewed, this section may be necessary. Previous work should be reviewed critically. See Chapter Eight for more information on writing a literature review.

Description of the Proposed Research

The description of the proposed research should be written for specialists in the field, not laypeople. This section is the heart of the proposal and is the primary concern of the technical reviewers. The technical aspects of the study must be completely covered. In general, be mindful of the following[1]:

1. Be realistic when designing the program of work. Overly optimistic notions of what the project can accomplish in 1, 2, or 3 years or of its effects on the world will only detract from the proposal's chances of being approved. Probably the comment most frequently made by reviewers is that the research plans should be scaled down to a more specific and more manageable project that will permit the approach to be evaluated and that, if successful, will form a sound basis for further work. In other words, your proposal should distinguish between long-range research goals and short-range objectives for which funding is being sought. Often it is best to begin this section with a short series of explicit statements listing each objective, in quantitative terms if possible.
2. If your first year must be spent developing an analytical method or laying groundwork, spell that out as Phase 1. Then at the end of the year you will be able to report that you have accomplished something and are ready to undertake Phase 2.
3. Be explicit about any assumptions or hypotheses the research method rests upon.
4. Be clear about the focus of the research. When defining the limits of the project, especially in exploratory or experimental work, it is helpful to pose the specific question or questions the project intends to answer.
5. Be as detailed as possible about the schedule of the proposed work. When will the first step be completed? When can subsequent steps be started? What must be done before what else, and what can be done at the same time? For complex projects, a calendar detailing the projected sequence and interrelationship of events often gives the sponsor assurance that the investigator is capable of careful step-by-step planning.
6. Be specific about the means of evaluating the data or the conclusions. Try to imagine the questions or objections of a hostile critic and show that the research plan anticipates them.
7. Be certain that the connection between the research objectives and the research method is evident. If a reviewer fails to see this connection, he or she will probably not give your proposal any further consideration. It is better to risk stating the obvious here than to risk the charge that you have not thought carefully enough about what your particular methods or approach can be expected to demonstrate.

Description of Relevant Institutional Resources

The nature of this section depends on your project, of course, but in general this section details the resources available to the proposed project and, if possible, shows why the sponsor should choose you and your institution for this particular research. Some relevant points may be the institution's demonstrated competence in the pertinent research area, its abundance of experts in related areas that may indirectly benefit the project, its supportive services that will directly benefit the project, and its unique or unusual research facilities or instruments available to the project.

List of References

The references should be prepared according to agency instructions. Many use citation methods described in widely distributed style manuals, such as the *AMA Manual of Style*.

Personnel

The personnel section is usually divided into two parts: a description of the proposed personnel arrangements and the biographical data sheets for all of the main contributors to the project. The description should state the number of people involved, their percentage of time involved, and their responsibilities during the project. Projects may involve people from multiple departments or colleges. It is important to clearly identify everyone's responsibilities in the project.

Biographical data sheets should be provided for all project personnel. These biosketches are generally no more than two pages and contain the following information:

- Educational background
- Employment history
- Recent publications
- Recent funded grants

Check agency guidelines to make sure you are providing the requested information.

Budget

The budget section includes a list of all budget items, their associated costs, and a budget justification. All are essential.

Budgets are typically divided into personnel, equipment, supplies, travel, and indirect costs. Other categories can be added as needed. It is important to "show your math" in the budget section. For example, you may present salary information for the principal investigator as follows: ½ time for 9 months @ $50,000 (9-month salary) = $25,000. This indicates how much time the principal investigator intends to spend on the project, how long he or she is going to work on the project, the nature of the base salary (9-month contract), and the total amount requested to pay this person.

It is important to present any costs absorbed by your institution. This is called *cost sharing*, and it demonstrates that your institution is also contributing to the project. While it is important to show cost-sharing figures, make sure they are presented clearly so as not to be confused with funds requested from the funding agency.

Indirect costs are shown as a separate category, usually as the last item before the grand total. Indirect costs are figured as a fixed percentage of the total direct costs. Because fixed indirect cost percentages change each year after negotiation with the federal government, proposal writers should consult their Office of Sponsored Projects, or a similar office, before calculating this part of their budget.

Table 9-2 contains a checklist of possible proposal budget items. Table 9-3 presents a sample budget section.

PROPOSALS TO PRIVATE FOUNDATIONS

Proposals to private foundations are generally more successful if they are preceded by an informal contact. This contact is usually a brief letter (not more than two pages) outlining the proposed project, suggesting why the foundation should be interested, and requesting an appointment to discuss it in further detail.

Most foundations have specific areas of interest for which they like to award funds. Make sure that the foundation is interested in the work you are proposing. Foundations rarely fund a project outside of their stated field of interest.

Table 9-2

EXAMPLES OF GRANT PROPOSAL BUDGET ITEMS

Salaries and Wages
Academic personnel
Research assistants
Stipends
Consultants (particularly statistical consultants)
Interviews
Computer programmer
Secretaries
Clerk-typists
Editorial assistants
Technicians
Subjects
Hourly personnel
Staff benefits
Salary increases in proposals that extend into a new year
Vacation accrual and/or use

Equipment
Fixed equipment
Movable equipment
Office equipment
Equipment installation

Materials and Supplies
Office supplies
Communications
Test materials
Questionnaire forms
Duplication materials
Animals
Animal care
Laboratory supplies
Glassware
Chemicals
Electronic supplies
Report materials and supplies

Travel
Administrative
Field work
Professional meetings
Travel for consultation
Consultants' travel
Subsistence
Automobile rental
Aircraft rental
Ship rental

Services
Computer use
Duplication services (reports, etc)
Publication costs
Photographic services
Service contracts

Other
Space rental
Alterations and renovations
Purchase of periodicals and books
Patient reimbursement
Tuition and fees (training grants)
Hospitalization
Page charges
Subcontracts

Indirect Costs

Table 9-3

SAMPLE BUDGET

Budget Period: July 1, 2001 to June 30, 2002

SALARIES	Sponsor	ABC University
Senior Personnel		
A.B. Charles, principal investigator		
9 months academic year—20%	$5494	$5494
2 months summer—100%	$12,208	
D.E. Frank, co-investigator		
9 months academic year—10%	$4000	
Consultant		
G.H. Iknowstats, statistical consultant		
9 months academic year—5%		$3250
Graduate Assistants		
9 months—50% (2)	$24,750	
TOTAL SALARIES	$46,452	$8,744
BENEFITS		
Faculty 22%, graduate students 1%	$5021	$1209
TOTAL BENEFITS	$5021	$1209
EQUIPMENT		
Super-duper laser device	$5300	
Super-duper laser device maintenance contract		$500
TOTAL EQUIPMENT	$5300	$500
SUPPLIES AND MATERIALS		
Electronic components	$3400	
Photographic materials	$2375	
Chemicals	$1250	
TOTAL SUPPLIES AND MATERIALS	$7025	
TRAVEL		
Airfare to ABC meeting	$300	
Hotel room (2 nights @ $100/night)	$200	
Subsistence (2 days @ $52/day)	$104	
TOTAL TRAVEL	$604	

Table 9-3 (Continued)		
OTHER DIRECT COSTS	Sponsor	ABC University
Publication costs	$750	
Telephone, fax, and postage	$700	
TOTAL OTHER DIRECT COSTS	$1450	
TOTAL DIRECT COSTS	$65,852	$10,453
INDIRECT COSTS		
Calculated at 50%	$30,276	$4,977
TOTAL BUDGET	$96,128	$15,430

The initial letter of inquiry should[1]:

1. Demonstrate that the investigator is acquainted with the work and purpose of the particular foundation being approached and point out a clear connection between it and the proposed project (form letters do not accomplish this).
2. Discuss the significance or uniqueness of the project. Who will benefit? Who cares about the results? What difference will it make if the project is not funded?
3. Give enough indication of step-by-step planning to show that the project has been thought through and that pitfalls have been anticipated.
4. Demonstrate your grasp of the subject and your credentials to undertake the project.
5. Emphasize at the same time that this is a preliminary inquiry, not a formal proposal, and that you will either send further details if the foundation wishes, or, better yet, will visit the foundation to discuss the project in depth. It is unnecessary to include a detailed budget in the preliminary inquiry, although an overall cost estimate should be mentioned.

A good letter, then, might begin something like the following[1]:

"Because of the interest the _____ Foundation has shown in _____, I am writing to solicit its support for a project that will _____."

A few sentences describing the program, the institution, and the need for and uniqueness of the project should follow this. The body of the letter should consist of three or four paragraphs that give the context or background of the project, its scope and methodology, the time required for its completion, the institutional commitments, and any special capabilities that will ensure the project's success. A separate paragraph might be given to some of the major categories of the proposed budget, including a rounded total direct cost estimate and mention of any matching fund or cost-sharing arrangements, either in dollars or in-kind contributions.

The last paragraph could be written as follows: "If the _____ Foundation is interested in learning more about this program, I will be happy to travel to _____ to discuss it in detail, or to submit a full proposal outlining my plans. My phone number in _____ is (__) _____ at work, and (__) _____ at home. I look forward to hearing from you soon."

In directories and other general sources of information, foundations often indicate their areas of interests in such broad terms that the investigator may not be able to determine with any confidence whether his or her project will interest them. More detailed guidance can be gleaned, however, from the foundation's annual reports and from the list of projects that the foundation has actually supported. In general, foundations are interested in innovative projects that are[1]:

- Relevant to pressing national or regional problems
- Relevant to new methods in education
- Capable of serving as models or stimuli for further or related work in its general area
- Capable of continuation after the end of the funding period without further assistance from the foundation
- Not eligible for funding by governmental agencies or the investigator's own institution

The letter of inquiry should highlight whichever of these characteristics best fits the project at hand.

DEALING WITH SHORT DEADLINES

Preparation of grant proposals should be planned out over months or years. Usually they are not and are often prepared as a deadline looms near. If you find yourself in this situation (as I often do), consider the following[1]:

1. Start (do not finish) with the sponsor's guidelines. Mark them as you study, noting such things as deadline (for mailing or arrival), number of copies, where to mail, and so on. Look for such requirements as the collection of institutional data that, were it left to last, could not be gathered. The guidelines will also likely specify certain topics or questions that must be addressed. If you can reasonably say anything at all on these topics, you should use the sponsor's exact phrases as your headings. You may even wish to borrow some of the language of the guidelines if it fits naturally into the framework of your proposal. If the sponsor is looking for "transdisciplinary" approaches to the problem, you would do well to use that term rather than "interdisciplinary" or "interdepartmental" to describe the same activities.
2. After you have studied the guidelines, if there are sections that are either too vague or too specific for comfort or convenience, check with the project representative to see if he or she has a clarification. If he or she does not, he or she may call the appropriate program officer at the agency for you or give you the number of the person to call. In either event, two ends will be served: the project representative will be alerted to your intentions to submit, and the information you will receive will help further focus the task of preparing a rush proposal.
3. Break the proposal up into small and simple subsections, especially if more than one person will be writing. Give each subsection headings and subheadings (referring again to the guidelines), and write slavishly to this outline. Using subheadings liberally will not only help you organize your material but will also guide reviewers through your perhaps not altogether flawlessly organized narrative. For facilitating last-minute corrections in the typed copy, start new sections and major subsections on new pages, and do not number pages, except lightly in pencil, until the last step.
4. Compare your budget and your text to ensure that for every cost figure a corresponding activity is mentioned and justified in the text.
5. Pay special attention to the abstract. Having rushed through the narrative, you will find that careful construction of the abstract will serve as both a summary of what you intend to do and a check on whether you have omitted any essential topics.

WHY PROPOSALS ARE REJECTED

Proposals are rejected for many reasons; however, some of the more common ones are[2]:

1. The problem is not of sufficient importance or is unlikely to produce any new or useful information.
2. The proposed research is based on a hypothesis that rests on insufficient evidence, is doubtful, or is unsound.

3. The problem is more complex than the investigator realizes.

4. The problem has only local significance, is one of production or control, or otherwise fails to fall sufficiently and clearly within the general field of health-related research.

5. The problem is scientifically premature and warrants, at most, only a pilot study.

6. The research as proposed is overly involved, with too many elements under simultaneous investigation.

7. The description of the nature and significance of the research leaves the proposal nebulous, diffuse, and without a clear research aim.

8. The proposed tests, methods, or scientific procedures are unsuited to the stated objective.

9. The description of the approach is too nebulous, diffuse, and lacking in clarity to permit adequate evaluation.

10. The overall design of the study has not been carefully thought out.

11. The statistical aspects of the approach have not been given sufficient consideration.

12. The approach lacks scientific imagination.

13. The controls are either inadequately conceived or inadequately described.

14. The material the investigator proposes to use is unsuited to the objective of the study or is difficult to obtain.

15. The number of observations is unsuitable.

16. The equipment contemplated is outmoded or otherwise unsuitable.

17. The investigator does not have adequate experience or training for this research.

18. The investigator appears to be unfamiliar with recent pertinent literature or methods.

19. The investigator's previously published work in this field does not inspire confidence.

20. The investigator proposes to rely too heavily on insufficiently experienced associates.

21. The investigator is spreading him- or herself too thin; he or she will be more productive if he or she concentrates on fewer projects.

22. The investigator needs more liaisons with colleagues in this field or in collateral fields.

23. The requirements for equipment or personnel are unrealistic.

24. It appears that other responsibilities would prevent devotion of sufficient time and attention to this research.

25. The institutional setting is unfavorable.

26. Previous research grants to the investigator are adequate in scope and amount to cover the proposed research.

Although this information is somewhat old, its applicability remains true today. Likewise, I have been unable to locate a source that provides as much detail.

REFERENCES

1. Thackrey D. Proposal Writer's Guide. University of Michigan. Available at: http://www.research.umich.edu/research/proposals/proposal_dev/pwg/pwg/complete.html. Accessed February 14, 2001.

2. Allen EM. Why are research grant applications disapproved? Characteristic shortcomings of rejected applications to the NIH are described. *Science.* 1960;132:1532-1534.

RECOMMENDED READING

Bauer DG. *The "How To" Grants Manual.* 2nd ed. New York: Macmillan Publishing Co; 1988.

Borland A, Margolin JE. *Foundation Center's User Friendly Guide: Grant Seekers' Guide to Research Resources.* New York: The Center; 1990.

Lefforts R. *Getting a Grant in the 1990s: How to Write Successful Grant Proposals.* New York: Prentice Hall Press; 1990.

Rice JB. *Applying for Research Funding: Getting Started and Getting Funded.* Thousand Oaks, Calif: Sage Publications; 1995.

Chapter Ten

Teaching Athletic Training Students About Research

"Read not to contradict and refute, nor to accept and take for granted, but to weigh and consider." —Sir Francis Bacon

Research is our good friend. It should be treated with due respect and incorporated into our lives as with any good friend. Just as we want our children to come to know a good family friend, we want our students to know research.

We need to teach our students how to do research and become scholarly practitioners. The degree to which we expose students to research depends on their level of preparation (ie, undergraduate vs. graduate), although it cannot be reinforced enough. Introduction of research into our curricula helps reinforce the following clinically relevant skills[1]:

1. Students learn how to use and understand clinically related instrumentation.
2. Students learn the scientific method and how to use it for clinical problem solving.
3. Students learn to appreciate research early in their preparation, and it will be a part of their clinical problem solving toolkit from the very beginning.
4. Students will be better prepared to contribute to the knowledge base through presentation and publication of their research findings (from original research papers to case reports).
5. Students will develop a life-long appreciation for the scientific method and scholarly problem-solving methods.

TEACHING RESEARCH TO UNDERGRADUATE STUDENTS

Students can be introduced to research and scholarship the minute they step on campus. Many athletic training students start their freshman year with an Introduction to (fill in the blank) class. Often, this is an Introduction to Allied Health Professions or the like. Students could have assignments in which they are required to find literature in the library (or online if you prefer) that is relevant to the profession. This involves use of electronic databases such as MEDLINE and Sport Discus. Yes, I am recommending that freshmen learn to do MEDLINE searches! Reinforcing to students that this is where new information is found and giving them the skills to locate this information are good starting points. Next, students must be able to find their way around a professional journal.

Incorporating assignments in the Introduction to Allied Health Professions (or similar) course that require students to locate information within journal articles helps them become comfortable. Ask students to answer specific questions about the journal article such as, "What is the purpose of the study?" "How many subjects were used in the study?" "What kind of subjects were used (eg, young or old, sedentary or active, men or women, etc)?" "What did the author(s) measure?" "What did the author(s) conclude?" and "What did you learn by reading this article?" Introduction to the scientific method and the concept of critical thinking can also be included in the freshman year.

The sophomore year is different at different institutions. Some students are selected for the professional component of the athletic training program after their freshman year and begin clinical instruction as a sophomore. In other programs, admittance into the professional component and clinical instruction does not begin until the junior year. Regardless, sophomores are ready to begin incorporating research into their classes and clinical experiences, if appropriate. Using research findings to support clinical decisions must begin as soon as the students are asked to formulate clinical decisions. As the students begin to take classes germane to athletic training, they should be required to find literature relevant to the topics discussed and write abstracts on the papers they read. Taking a basic research design class could occur as soon as the sophomore year. Students could be introduced to and asked to sit in on journal club meetings. Participation in journal club discussions should be encouraged. Juniors and seniors should be active participants in these discussions and positively model the research culture to sophomores. Instructors should also include required journal reading in addition to textbooks as a part of class. Students must understand at a very early stage of their formal education that textbooks are not the only source for information. They must learn that the most current and specialized information is in journal articles.

Juniors are ready to begin incorporating the principles of research into everything they do. They should continue with the skills learned as sophomores, including writing abstracts as a part of classes and participating in the journal club; however, they should now be expected to be able to find support for their clinical decisions in the literature. They must also come to understand that not all clinical activities can be directly supported in the literature. Some clinical decisions can be supported by the literature; some must be supported by good old-fashioned logic. Juniors need to be able to appreciate when each is appropriate. Juniors ought to take a statistics class to learn about testing research hypotheses and understanding human variability. Writing literature-supported technique papers or case reports for classes helps juniors incorporate their knowledge of research into clinically relevant information. Finally, juniors should begin thinking about their senior theses or research projects. Formal proposals may be required at the end of the junior year.

Seniors should have a hands-on experience with the scientific method. Usually, this is accomplished in the form of a senior thesis or research project. Writing literature review papers is helpful to understanding what is written, but students cannot fully appreciate how new knowledge is created if they are not required to do it. The senior thesis or research project, coupled with case reports and technique papers, will make the students astute consumers of the literature as well as potential contributors. Seniors should take leadership roles in the journal club. They should lead discussions and be avid critics of the papers under discussion. They should be able to formulate appropriate generalizations from their readings. A clinical rotation in a research laboratory can reinforce the importance of research as a clinical tool.

The extent to which undergraduate students value research and use the literature to guide their decisions will be based largely on how that type of behavior is modeled. These behaviors must be encouraged and modeled in the classroom and, most importantly, in the clinic. If students do not see our practitioners incorporating research into their own decision-making, they will be less likely to use these skills when they become practitioners. Failure to do so weakens the profession. A profession that makes decisions based solely on intuition and information learned as a student is not a profession. In the end, patients benefit from practitioners with many problem-solving tools.

Undergraduate students at all levels should be encouraged to participate in research projects (Table 10-1). While participating, they can get a first hand experience of how research is conducted and begin to develop an appreciation of the work that goes into doing research. Important answers to important professional questions come only through hard work!

Table 10-1			
RESEARCH ACTIVITIES DURING EACH ACADEMIC YEAR			
Freshman Yr	Sophomore Yr	Junior Yr	Senior Yr
Locate professional journals	Introduce use of research findings	Continue writing abstracts in classes	Complete a senior thesis or research project
Find specific information within articles	Require abstracts of relevant papers as part of classes	Require research support of clinical decisions	Lead discussions in journal club
Introduce the scientific method	Basic research design class	Statistics class	Clinical rotation in research laboratory
Introduce concepts of critical thinking	Introduce to journal club	Participate in journal club	
	Include required journal article readings as part of classes	Develop proposals for senior thesis or research project	
		Write literature-supported technique papers or case reports	

TEACHING RESEARCH TO GRADUATE STUDENTS

Research becomes even more important for graduate students. One of the differentiating factors between an athletic trainer who has graduate education and one with an undergraduate education is the extent to which he or she understands research and integrates it into clinical practice.

The research experiences for masters and doctoral students should be somewhat different (more intense for doctoral students), but many of the same elements can be incorporated.

Masters Students

Masters students enjoy and struggle with the transition from a competency-based learning environment required to have general competence as an athletic trainer to more indepth, specialized learning. As such, research becomes a more important element in the learning process. Masters-level students should:

- Have a research/statistics class
- Have research integrated into all of their coursework
- Complete a thesis or research project, or minimally have some hands-on experience with the scientific method
- Participate in journal clubs
- Become avid consumers of the literature in their clinical decision-making capacities

Above all else, we need to teach our masters students to be scholarly practitioners. They need to use the literature to guide their practice, understand and properly apply generalizations from studies, and use good critical thinking skills.

Doctoral Students

Doctoral students should become experts in research, as this is an essential element in becoming a scholar. Doctoral students are the future scholars in the field. If they do not have a solid preparation in research, their ability to become scholars is minimized.

I suggest integrating the following activities into preparation of doctoral students:

1. Get them involved in research groups. They get a chance to see how ideas develop into studies and how studies develop into theory. They get to see scientists practicing their craft.
2. Spend time reviewing literature together. Find positive and negative aspects of papers. Assign students to "deconstruct" a paper. This paper deconstruction assignment encourages them to carefully evaluate everything about the paper. It is surprising how much students get out of this experience. They read literature in an entirely different way after an experience like this.
3. GITL! This phrase is commonly heard at Indiana State University and means Get In The Lab. Spending time "playing" with instruments and trying things out together help students really understand what the instruments measure.
4. Require students to write a real grant (not just ones for a grant writing class) and submit it to a funding agency. Even if it is an intramural grant, the experience is invaluable and is an essential tool for young scholars entering the academy.
5. Insist on scholarly behavior. Students learn the language of scholarship by practicing it often. Sweetly, but firmly, insist that students discuss professional matters from a scholarly perspective. Gossip and hearsay are verboten!
6. Make sure students have interactions with other scholars in the field and in other professions. Learning to talk about research with a diverse group of scholars is an important survival skill in the academy. This networking can also help them find jobs and develop research teams in the future.
7. If possible, have doctoral students help you mentor masters students who are working on theses or research projects. When a doctoral student completes his or her program, he or she may have to chair theses, dissertations, or research projects. It is best if they learn how to do that with their mentor and not on their own.
8. Require students to complete research and publish papers before their dissertation work. Students need to learn how studies build upon one another to develop theory. As a result, their research and writing skills will also be much better at dissertation time.
9. Spend a lot of time talking about ideas for research projects. Students need to learn that some ideas "dead end," some develop into viable studies, and many change drastically from conception to inception.
10. Encourage independent thinking. Spoon-feeding doctoral students benefits no one. They need to struggle with ideas, work through frustrations, and learn how to find answers for themselves. Doctoral students who do not learn how to find answers for themselves have missed out on one of the most important lessons they could learn, in my opinion.

The examples and suggestions used throughout this chapter are certainly not all-inclusive. I suggest sharing ideas with colleagues and adding your own ideas to this preliminary list. You can even write in the book if you want to.

REFERENCE

1. Deem JF, Gonzalez LS. Teaching research in the undergraduate curriculum: influencing student attitudes. *J Allied Health.* 1999;28:247-251.

Glossary

A-21: "Cost Principles for Educational Institutions," a circular published by the Federal Office of Management and Budget (OMB) that establishes the principles for determining the costs applicable to grants, contracts, and other government agreements with educational institutions (also known as Sponsored Projects).

AAALAC: American Association for the Accreditation of Lab Animal Care.

abuse-liable: pharmacological substances that have the potential for creating abusive dependency. Abuse-liable substances can include both illicit drugs (eg, heroin) and licit drugs (eg, methamphetamines).

academy: a society of scholars, scientists, or artists.

adjuvant therapy: therapy provided to enhance the effect of a primary therapy; auxiliary therapy.

adverse effect: an undesirable and unintended, although not necessarily unexpected, result of therapy or other intervention (eg, headache following a spinal tap or intestinal bleeding associated with aspirin therapy).

allocable costs: those allowable costs that actually benefit the grant or contract to which they are being charged.

allowable costs: those categories of costs that can be charged to a grant, such as salaries and equipment. Certain types of costs, such as the cost of alcoholic beverages, are not allowable and may not be charged to a contract or grant.

AMA: American Medical Association.

assent: agreement by an individual not competent to give legally valid informed consent (ie, a child or cognitively impaired person) to participate in research.

assurance: a formal written, binding commitment that is submitted to a federal agency in which an institution promises to comply with applicable regulations governing research with human subjects and stipulates the procedures through which compliance will be achieved (Federal Policy §___.103).

audit: a formal examination of an organization's or individual's accounts or financial situation. An audit may also include examination of compliance with applicable terms, laws, and regulations.

authorized institutional official: an officer of an institution with the authority to speak for and legally commit the institution to adherence to the requirements of the federal regulations regarding the involvement of human subjects in biomedical and behavioral research.

autonomy: personal capacity to consider alternatives, make choices, and act without undue influence or interference of others.

award: funds that have been obligated by a funding agency for a particular project.

basic science: (in athletic training context) controlled laboratory studies in the subdisciplines of exercise physiology, biomechanics, and motor behavior, among others, that relate to athletic training and sports medicine.

Belmont Report: a statement of basic ethical principles governing research involving human subjects issued by the National Commission for the Protection of Human Subjects in 1978.

beneficence: an ethical principle discussed in the Belmont Report that entails an obligation to protect persons from harm. The principle of beneficence can be expressed in two general rules: (1) do not harm and (2) protect from harm by maximizing possible benefits and minimizing possible risks of harm.

benefit: a valued or desired outcome; an advantage.

Broad Agency Announcement (BAA): an announcement of a federal agency's general research interests that invites proposals and specifies the general terms and conditions under which an award may be made.

budget: the detailed statement outlining estimated project costs to support work under a grant or contract.

budget period: the interval of time—usually 12 months—into which the project period is divided for budgetary and funding purposes.

CAS: Cost Accounting Standards.

case-control study: a study comparing persons with a given condition or disease (the cases) and persons without the condition or disease (the controls) with respect to antecedent factors (see also *retrospective studies*).

CDC: Centers for Disease Control and Prevention.

CFDA: Catalog of Federal Domestic Assistance.

CFR: Code of Federal Regulations.

challenge grant: a grant that provides monies in response to monies from other sources, usually according to a formula. A challenge grant may, for example, offer two dollars for every one that is obtained from a fund drive. The grant usually has a fixed upper limit and may have a challenge minimum below which no grant will be made. This form of grant is fairly common in the arts, humanities, and some other fields but is less common in the sciences. A challenge grant differs from a matching grant in at least one important respect: the amount of money that the recipient organization realizes from a challenge grant may vary widely, depending upon how successful that organization is in meeting the challenge. Matching grants usually award a clearly defined amount and require that a specified sum be obtained before any award is made.

children: persons who have not attained the legal age for consent to treatment or procedures involved in research, as determined under the applicable law of the jurisdiction in which the research will be conducted (45 CFR 46.401[a]).

clinical study: (in athletic training context) studies including assessment of the validity, reliability, and efficacy of clinical procedures, rehabilitation protocols, injury prevention programs, surgical techniques, and so on.

clinical trial: a controlled study involving human subjects designed to prospectively evaluate the safety and effectiveness of new drugs or devices or of behavioral interventions.

close out: the act of completing all internal procedures and sponsor requirements to terminate or complete a research project.

COGR: Council on Governmental Relations.

cohort: a group of subjects initially identified as having one or more characteristics in common who are followed over time. In social science research, this term may refer to any group of persons who are born at about the same time and share common historical or cultural experiences.

compensation: payment or medical care provided to subjects injured in research; does not refer to payment (remuneration) for participation in research (compare with *remuneration*).

competence: technically, a legal term used to denote capacity to act on one's own behalf; the ability to understand information presented, to appreciate the consequences of acting (or not acting) on that information, and to make a choice (see also *incompetence, incapacity*).

competing proposals: proposals that are submitted for the first time or unfunded proposals that are resubmitted; either must compete for research funds. Ongoing projects must compete again if the term of the original award has expired.

confidentiality: pertains to the treatment of information that an individual has disclosed in a relationship of trust with the expectation that it will not be divulged to others without permission in ways that are inconsistent with the understanding of the original disclosure.

consortium agreement: group of collaborative investigators/institutions; arrangement can be formalized with specified terms and conditions.

continuation project: applicable to grants and cooperative agreements only. A project approved for multiple-year funding, although funds are typically committed only 1 year at a time. At the end of the initial budget period, progress on the project is assessed. If satisfactory, an award is made for the next budget period, subject to the availability of funds. Continuation projects do not compete with new project proposals and are not subjected to peer review beyond the initial project approval.

contract[1]: a mechanism for procurement of a product or service with specific obligations for both sponsor and recipient. Typically, the sponsor specifies in detail a research topic and the methods for conducting the research, although some sponsors award contracts in response to unsolicited proposals.

contract[2]: an agreement; as used here, an agreement that a specific research activity will be performed at the request and under the direction of the agency providing the funds. Research performed under contract is more closely controlled by the agency than research performed under a grant (compare with *grant*).

contract/grant officer: a sponsor's designated individual who is officially responsible for the business management aspects of a particular grant, cooperative agreement, or contract. Serving as the counterpart to the business officer of the contractor/ grantee organization, the contract/ grant officer is responsible for all business management matters associated with the review, negotiation, award, and administration of a grant or contract and interprets the associated administration policies, regulations, and provisions.

contraindicated: disadvantageous, perhaps dangerous; a treatment that should not be used in certain individuals or conditions due to risks (eg, a drug may be contraindicated for pregnant women and persons with high blood pressure).

control(s): subject(s) used for comparison who are not given a treatment under study or who do not have a given condition, background, or risk factor that is the object of study. Control conditions may be concurrent (occurring more or less simultaneously with the condition under study) or historical (preceding the condition under study). When the present condition of subjects is compared with their own condition on a prior regimen or treatment, the study is considered historically controlled.

cooperative agreement: an award similar to a grant, but in which the sponsor's staff may be actively involved in proposal preparation and anticipates having substantial involvement in research activities once the award has been made.

correlation coefficient: a statistical index of the degree of relationship between two variables. Values of correlation coefficients range from -1.00 through 0.00 to +1.00. A correlation coefficient of 0.00 indicates no relationship between the variables. Correlations approaching -1.00 or +1.00 indicate strong relationships between the variables; however, causal inferences about the relationship between two variables can never be made on the basis of correlation coefficients, no matter how strong a relationship is indicated.

cost accounting standards (CAS): federally mandated accounting standards intended to ensure uniformity in budgeting and spending funds.

cost-reimbursement-type contract/grant: a contract/grant for which the sponsor pays for the full costs incurred in the conduct of the work up to an agreed-upon amount.

cost-sharing: a general term, used as a noun or adjective, that can describe virtually any type of arrangement in which more than one party supports research, equipment acquisition, demonstration projects, programs, institutions. Example: a university receives a grant for a project estimated to have a total cost of $100,000. The sponsor agrees to pay 75% ($75,000) and the university agrees to pay 25% ($25,000). The $25,000 is the cost-sharing component.

CRADA or CRDA: Cooperative Research and Development Agreement.

cross-over design: a type of clinical trial in which each subject experiences, at different times, both the experimental and control therapy. For example, half of the subjects might be randomly assigned first to the control group and then to the experimental intervention, while the other half would have the sequence reversed.

data and safety monitoring board: a committee of scientists, physicians, statisticians, and others that collects and analyzes data during the course of a clinical trial to monitor for adverse effects and other trends (such as an indication that one treatment is significantly better than another, particularly when one arm of the trial involves a placebo control) that would warrant modification or termination of the trial or notification of subjects about new information that might affect their willingness to continue in the trial.

debriefing: giving subjects previously undisclosed information about the research project following completion of their participation in research. (Note that this usage, which occurs within the behavioral sciences, departs from standard English, in which debriefing is obtaining rather than imparting information.)

Declaration of Helsinki: a code of ethics for clinical research approved by the World Medical Association in 1964 and widely adopted by medical associations in various countries. It was revised in 1975 and 1989.

DED: Department of Education.

deficit: expenditures exceed available funds.

dependent variables: the outcomes that are measured in an experiment. Dependent variables are expected to change as a result of an experimental manipulation of the independent variable(s).

descriptive study: any study that is not truly experimental (eg, quasi-experimental studies, correlational studies, record reviews, case histories, and observational studies).

DHHS: Department of Health and Human Services.

direct costs: clearly identifiable costs related to a specific project. General categories of direct costs include but are not limited to salaries and wages, fringe benefits, supplies, contractual services, travel and communication, equipment, and computer use.

donation: transfer of equipment, money, goods, services, and property with or without specifications as to its use. Sometimes a donation is used to designate contributions that are made with more specific intent than is usually the case with a gift, but the two terms are often used interchangeably (see also *gift*).

double-masked design: a study design in which neither the investigators nor the subjects know the treatment group assignments of individual subjects. Sometimes referred to as "double-blind."

educational research: (in athletic training context) a broad category ranging from basic surveys to detailed athletic training/sports medicine curricular development. Generally includes assessment of student learning, teaching effectiveness (didactic or clinical), educational materials, and curricular development.

emancipated minor: a legal status conferred upon persons who have not yet attained the age of legal competency as defined by state law (for such purposes as consenting to medical care), but who are entitled to treatment as if they had by virtue of assuming adult responsibilities such as being self-supporting and not living at home, marriage, or procreation (see also *mature minor*).

encumbrance: funds that have been set aside or "claimed" for projected expenses pending actual expenditure of the funds.

endowment: a fund, usually in the form of an income-generating investment, established to provide long-term support for faculty/research positions (eg, endowed chair).

epidemiology: a scientific discipline that studies the factors determining the causes, frequency, and distribution of diseases in a community or given population.

epistemology: the study or theory of the nature and grounds of knowledge, especially with reference to its limits and validity.

equitable: fair or just; used in the context of selection of subjects to indicate that the benefits and burdens of research are fairly distributed (Federal Policy §___.111[a][3]).

ethics advisory board: an interdisciplinary group that advises the secretary of the Department of Health and Human Services (HHS), on general policy matters and on research proposals (or classes of proposals) that pose ethical problems.

ethnographic research: ethnography is the study of people and their culture. Ethnographic research, also called fieldwork, involves observation of and interaction with the persons or group being studied in the group's own environment, often for long periods of time (see also *fieldwork*).

expanded availability: policy and procedure that permits individuals who have serious or life-threatening diseases for which there are no alternative therapies to have access to investigational drugs and devices that may be beneficial to them.

expedited review: review of proposed research by the IRB chair or a designated voting member or group of voting members rather than by the entire IRB. Federal rules permit expedited review for certain kinds of research involving no more than minimal risk and for minor changes in approved research (Federal Policy §___.110).

experimental: term often used to denote a therapy (drug, device, procedure) that is unproven or not yet scientifically validated with respect to safety and efficacy. A procedure may be considered "experimental" without necessarily being part of a formal study (research) to evaluate its usefulness (see also *research*).

experimental study: a true experimental study is one in which subjects are randomly assigned to groups that experience carefully controlled interventions manipulated by the experimenter according to a strict logic allowing causal inference about the effects of the interventions under investigation (see also *quasi-experimental study*).

expiration date: the date signifying the end of the performance period, as indicated on the notice of grant award.

extension: an additional period of time given by the sponsor to an organization for the completion of work on an approved grant or contract. An extension allows previously allocated funds to be spent after the original expiration date.

facilities and administrative (F&A) costs: costs that are incurred for common or joint objectives and, therefore, cannot be identified readily and specifically with a particular sponsored project, an instructional activity, or any other institutional activity. F&A costs are synonymous with indirect costs.

false negative: when a test wrongly shows an effect or condition to be absent (eg, that a woman is not pregnant when, in fact, she is).

false positive: when a test wrongly shows an effect or condition to be present (eg, that a woman is pregnant when, in fact, she is not).

Federal Policy (The): the federal policy that provides regulations for the involvement of human subjects in research. The policy applies to all research involving human subjects conducted, supported, or otherwise subject to regulation by any federal department or agency that takes appropriate administrative action to make the policy applicable to such research. Currently, 16 federal agencies have adopted the Federal Policy (also known as the Common Rule).

fieldwork: behavioral, social, or anthropological research involving the study of persons or groups in their own environment and without manipulation for research purposes (distinguished from laboratory or controlled settings) (see also *ethnographic research*).

final report: the final technical or financial report required by the sponsor to complete a research project.

fixed price (FP) contract/grant: a contract/grant for which one party pays the other party a predetermined price, regardless of actual costs, for services rendered. Quite often this is a fee-for-service agreement.

FOIA: Freedom of Information Act.

fringe benefits: employee benefits paid by the employer (eg, FICA, Workers' Compensation, Withholding Tax, Insurance, etc).

full board review: review of proposed research at a convened meeting at which a majority of the membership of the IRB is present, including at least one member whose primary concerns are in non-scientific areas. For the research to be approved, it must receive the approval of a majority of those members present at the meeting (Federal Policy §___.108).

funding cycle: range of time during which proposals are accepted and reviewed and funds are awarded. If a sponsor has standing proposal review committees (or boards) that meet at specified times during the year, application deadlines are set to correspond with those meetings. For some sponsors, if proposals are received too late to be considered in the current funding cycle, they may be held over for the next review.

gift: gifts and bequests are awards given with few or no conditions specified. Gifts may be provided to establish an endowment or to provide direct support for existing programs. Frequently, gifts are used to support developing programs for which other funding is not available. The unique flexibility, or lack of restrictions, makes gifts attractive sources of support (see also *donation*).

GPG: Grant Proposal Guide for the National Science Foundation.

grant: a type of financial assistance awarded to an organization for the conduct of research or other programs as specified in an approved proposal. A grant, as opposed to a cooperative agreement, is used whenever the awarding office anticipates no substantial programmatic involvement with the recipient during the performance of the activities.

grant: financial support provided for research study designed and proposed by the principal investigator(s). The granting agency exercises no direct control over the conduct of approved research supported by a grant (compare with *contract*).

guardian: an individual who is authorized under applicable state or local law to give permission on behalf of a child for general medical care (45 CFR 46.402 [3]).

historical controls: control subjects (followed at some time in the past or for whom data are available through records) who are used for comparison with subjects being treated concurrently. The study is considered historically controlled when the present condition of the subjects is compared with their own condition on a prior regimen or treatment.

human subjects: individuals whose physiologic or behavioral characteristics and responses are the object of study in a research project. Under federal regulations, human subjects are defined as living individual(s) about whom an investigator conducting research obtains (1) data through intervention or interaction with the individual or (2) identifiable private information (Federal Policy §___.102[f]).

IACUC: Institutional Animal Care and Use Committee.

IBC: Institutional Biosafety Committee.

iconoclast: one who attacks traditional ideas or institutions.

IFB: invitation for bid.

incapacity: refers to a person's mental status and means the inability to understand information presented, to appreciate the consequences of acting (or not acting) on that information, and to make a choice. Often used as a synonym for incompetence (see also *incompetence*).

incompetence: technically, a legal term meaning inability to manage one's own affairs. Often used as a synonym for incapacity (see also *incapacity*).

incremental funding: a method of funding contracts that provides specific spending limits below the total estimated costs. These limits may be exceeded only at the contractor's own risk. Each increment is, in essence, a funding action.

independent variables: the conditions of an experiment that are systematically manipulated by the investigator.

indirect cost rate: the rate, expressed as a percentage of a base amount (modified total direct cost [MTDC]), established by negotiation with the cognizant federal agency on the basis of the institution's projected costs for the year and distributed as prescribed in OMB Circular A-21. At UCLA, indirect costs are applied to a MTDC base. The indirect cost rate is charged on a set of direct costs known as an indirect cost base.

indirect costs: costs related to expenses incurred in conducting or supporting research or other externally funded activities but not directly attributable to a specific project. General categories of indirect costs include general administration (accounting, payroll, purchasing, etc), sponsored project administration, plant operation and maintenance, library expenses, departmental administration expenses, depreciation or use allowance for buildings and equipment, and student administration and services (see also *facilities* and *administrative costs*).

informed consent: a person's voluntary agreement, based upon adequate knowledge and understanding of relevant information, to participate in research or to undergo a diagnostic, therapeutic, or preventive procedure. In giving informed consent, subjects may not waive or appear to waive any of their legal rights or release or appear to release the investigator, the sponsor, the institution, or agents thereof from liability for negligence (Federal Policy §116; 21 CFR 50.20 and 50.25).

in-kind: contributions or assistance in a form other than money. Equipment, materials, or services of recognized value that are offered in lieu of cash.

institutional review board (IRB): a specially constituted review body established or designated by an entity to protect the welfare of human subjects recruited to participate in biomedical or behavioral research (Federal Policy §§___.102[g], ___.108, ___.109).

institutionalized: confined, either voluntarily or involuntarily (eg, a hospital, prison, or nursing home).

interim funding: authorization to expend funds on a project to a specified limit before the award document has been received from the sponsor.

investigator: in clinical trials, an individual who actually conducts an investigation [21 CFR 312.3]. Any interventions (eg, drugs) involved in the study are administered to subjects under the immediate direction of the investigator (see also *principal investigator*).

investigator-initiated proposal: a proposal submitted to a sponsor that is not in response to an RFP, RFA, or a specific program announcement.

invitation for bid (IFB): a solicitation issued to prospective bidders. An IFB describes what is required and how the bidders will be evaluated. Award is based on the lowest bid. Negotiations are not conducted.

IRB: Institutional Review Board.

justice: an ethical principle discussed in the Belmont Report requiring fairness in distribution of burdens and benefits; often expressed in terms of treating persons of similar circumstances or characteristics similarly.

key personnel: the personnel considered to be of primary importance to the successful conduct of a research project. The term usually applies to the senior members of the project staff.

knowledge: the state or fact of knowing. Familiarity, awareness, or understanding gained through experience or study. The sum or range of what has been perceived, discovered, or learned.

legally authorized representative: a person authorized either by statute or by court appointment to make decisions on behalf of another person. In human subjects research, an individual or judicial or other body authorized under applicable law to consent on behalf of a prospective subject to the subject's participation in the procedure(s) involved in the research (Federal Policy §___.102[c]).

limitation of cost (LOC): a mandatory clause for cost-reimbursement-type contracts. Under the clause, the sponsor is not obligated to reimburse the contractor for costs in excess of the stated amount. The contractor, however, is not obligated to continue performance once expenses reach the stated amount.

longitudinal study: a study designed to follow subjects forward through time.

masked study designs: study designs comparing two or more interventions in which either the investigators, the subjects, or some combination thereof do not know the treatment group assignments of individual subjects. Sometimes called "blind" study designs (see also *double-masked design, single-masked design*).

matching grant: a grant that requires a specified portion of the cost of a supported item of equipment or project be obtained from other sources. The required match may be more or less than the amount of the grant. Some matching grants require that the additional funds be obtained from sources outside the recipient organization. Many matching grants are paid in installments, the payments coinciding with the attainment of prespecified levels of additional funding (see also *challenge grant*).

mature minor: Someone who has not reached adulthood (as defined by state law) but who may be treated as an adult for certain purposes (eg, consenting to medical care). Note that a mature minor is not necessarily an emancipated minor (see also *emancipated minor*).

minimal risk: a risk is minimal when the probability and magnitude of harm or discomfort anticipated in the proposed research are not greater, in and of themselves, than those ordinarily encountered in daily life or during the performance of routine physical or psychological examinations or tests (Federal Policy §___.102[i]). For example, the risk of drawing a small amount of blood from a healthy individual for research purposes is no greater than the risk of doing so as part of a routine physical examination. The definition of minimal risk for research involving prisoners differs somewhat from that given for noninstitutionalized adults. (*see* 45 CFR 46.303[d] and Guidebook Chapter 6, Section E, "Prisoners.")

monitoring: the collection and analysis of data as the project progresses to assure the appropriateness of the research, its design, and subject protections.

NAS: National Academy of Sciences.

NASA: National Aeronautics and Space Administration.

NCURA: National Council of University Research Administrators.

NEI: National Eye Institute (NIH).

new and competing proposals: proposals that are submitted for the first time or ongoing projects that must recompete for funding prior to expiration of the original award.

new award: an award not previously awarded or a renewal or continuation award treated as a new award by the sponsor and given a new agency number.

NHLBI: National Heart, Lung, and Blood Institute (NIH).

NIA: National Institute on Aging (NIH).

NIAID: National Institute of Allergy and Infectious Diseases (NIH).

NIAMS: National Institute of Arthritis and Musculoskeletal and Skin Diseases (NIH).

NIH: National Institutes of Health.

NIMH: National Institute of Mental Health (NIH).

NINDS: National Institute of Neurological Disorders and Stroke (NIH).

NLM: National Library of Medicine.

no cost time extension: an extension of the period of performance beyond the expiration date to allow the principal investigator to finish a project. Usually, no additional costs are provided.

nonaffiliated member: member of an IRB who has no ties to the parent institution, its staff, or faculty. This individual is usually from the local community (eg, minister, business person, attorney, teacher, homemaker).

nontherapeutic research: research that has no likelihood or intent of producing a diagnostic, preventive, or therapeutic benefit to the current subjects, although it may benefit subjects with a similar condition in the future.

normal volunteers: volunteer subjects used to study normal physiology and behavior or who do not have the condition under study in a particular protocol, used as comparisons with subjects who do have the condition. "Normal" may not mean normal in all respects. For example, patients with broken legs (if not on medication that will affect the results) may serve as normal volunteers in studies of metabolism, cognitive development, and the like. Similarly, patients with heart disease but without diabetes may be the "normals" in a study of diabetes complicated by heart disease.

notice of grant award: legally binding document that serves as a notification to the recipient and others that a grant or cooperative agreement has been made, contains or references all terms of the award, and documents the obligation of funds.

NSF: National Science Foundation.

null hypothesis: the proposition, to be tested statistically, that the experimental intervention has "no effect," meaning that the treatment and control groups will not differ as a result of the intervention. Investigators usually hope that the data will demonstrate some effect from the intervention, thereby allowing the investigator to reject the null hypothesis.

Nuremberg Code: a code of research ethics developed during the trials of Nazi war criminals following World War II and widely adopted as a standard during the 1950s and 1960s for protecting human subjects.

observation/informational studies: (in athletic training context) includes studies involving surveys, questionnaires, and descriptive programs, among others, that relate to athletic training and sports medicine.

OMB: Office of Management and Budget.

open design: an experimental design in which both the investigator(s) and the subject(s) know the treatment group(s) to which subjects are assigned.

OPRR: Office for Protection from Research Risks (DHHS).

parallelism: (grammatical) similar ideas are expressed in a similar, or parallel, fashion.

paternalism: making decisions for others against or apart from their wishes with the intent of doing them good.

peer review: a system using reviewers who are the professional equals of the principal investigator or program director who is to be responsible for directing or conducting the proposed project. It is a form of objective review. Peer review is legislatively mandated in some programs and is administratively required in other programs.

permission: the agreement of parent(s) or guardian(s) to the participation of their child or ward in research (45 CFR 46.402[c]).

person: (grammatical) the form of a verb or a pronoun that indicates whether a person is speaking (first person), is spoken to (second person), or is spoken about (third person).

PI: principal investigator.

placebo: a chemically inert substance given in the guise of medicine for its psychologically suggestive effect; used in controlled clinical trials to determine whether improvement and side effects may reflect imagination or anticipation rather than the actual power of a drug.

preclinical investigation: laboratory and animal studies designed to test the mechanisms, safety, and efficacy of an intervention prior to its applications to humans.

preproposal: a brief description, usually 2 to 10 pages, of research plans and estimated budget that is sometimes submitted to determine the interest of a particular sponsor prior to submission of a formal proposal. Also termed *preliminary proposal.*

principal investigator: the individual responsible for the conduct of research or other activity described in a proposal for an award; the scientist or scholar with primary responsibility for the design and conduct of a research project (see also *investigator*).

prisoner: an individual involuntarily confined in a penal institution, including persons (1) sentenced under a criminal or civil statue; (2) detained pending arraignment, trial, or sentencing; and (3) detained in other facilities (eg, for drug detoxification or treatment of alcoholism) under statutes or commitment procedures providing such alternatives to criminal prosecution or incarceration in a penal institution (45 CFR 46.303[c]).

privacy: control over the extent, timing, and circumstances of sharing one's self (physically, behaviorally, or intellectually) with others.

proband: the person whose case serves as the stimulus for the study of other members of the family to identify the possible genetic factors involved in a given disease, condition, or characteristic.

profession: an occupation requiring training and specialized study.

program/project officer: a sponsor's designated individual officially responsible for the technical, scientific, or programmatic aspects of a particular grant, cooperative agreement, or contract. Serving as the counterpart to the principal investigator/project director of the grantee/contractor organization, the program/project officer deals with the grantee/contractor organization staff to assure programmatic progress.

progress report: periodic, scheduled report required by the sponsor that summarizes research progress to date. Technical, fiscal, and invention reports may be required.

project period (PP): the total time for which support of a project has been programmatically approved. A project period may consist of one or more budget periods (see also *budget period*).

prophylactic: preventive or protective; a drug, vaccine, regimen, or device designed to prevent or provide protection against a given disease or disorder.

proposal: an application for funding that contains all information necessary to describe project plans, staff capabilities, and funds requested. Formal proposals are officially approved and submitted by an organization in the name of a principal investigator.

prospective studies: studies designed to observe outcomes or events that occur subsequent to the identification of the group of subjects to be studied. Prospective studies need not involve manipulation or intervention but may be purely observational or involve only the collection of data.

protocol: the formal design or plan of an experiment or research activity; specifically, the plan submitted to an IRB for review and to an agency for research support. The protocol includes a description of the research design or methodology to be employed, the eligibility requirements for prospective subjects and controls, the treatment regimen(s), and the proposed methods of analysis that will be performed on the collected data.

quasi-experimental study: a study that is similar to a true experimental study except that it lacks random assignments of subjects to treatment groups (see also *experimental study*).

random, random assignment, randomization, randomized: assignment of subjects to different treatments, interventions, or conditions according to chance rather than systematically (ie, as dictated by the standard or usual response to their condition, history, or prognosis, or according to demographic characteristics). Random assignment of subjects to conditions is an essential element of experimental research because it makes the probability more likely that differences observed between subject groups are the result of the experimental intervention.

rebudget: the act of amending the budget by moving funds from one category or line item to another (see also *budget adjustment*).

remuneration: payment for participation in research (Note: It is wise to confine use of the term "compensation" to payment or provision of care for research-related injuries.) (compare with *compensation*).

renewal: applicable to grants and cooperative agreements only. A competitively reviewed proposal requesting additional funds extending the scope of work beyond the current project period.

request for application (RFA): announcement that indicates the availability of funds for a topic of specific interest to a sponsor. Proposals submitted in response to RFAs generally result in the award of a grant. Specific grant announcements may be published in the Federal Register and/or specific sponsor publications (see also *broad agency announcements*).

request for proposal (RFP): announcement that specifies a topic of research, methods to be used, product to be delivered, and appropriate applicants sought. Proposals submitted in response to RFPs generally result in the award of a contract.

research: a systematic investigation (ie, the gathering and analysis of information) designed to develop or contribute to generalizable knowledge (Federal Policy §___.102[d]).

respect for persons: an ethical principle discussed in the Belmont Report requiring that individual autonomy be respected and that persons with diminished autonomy be protected.

retrospective studies: research conducted by reviewing records from the past (eg, birth and death certificates, medical records, school records, or employment records) or by obtaining information about past events elicited through interviews or surveys. Case control studies are an example of this type of research.

review (of research): the concurrent oversight of research on a periodic basis by an IRB. In addition to at least the annual reviews mandated by the federal regulations, reviews may, if deemed appropriate, also be conducted on a continuous or periodic basis (Federal Policy §___.108[e]).

risk: the probability of harm or injury (physical, psychological, social, or economic) occurring as a result of participation in a research study. Both the probability and magnitude of possible harm may vary from minimal to significant. Federal regulations define only "minimal risk" (see also *minimal risk*).

risk management: managing resources wisely, protecting clients from harm, and safeguarding assets.

salaries and wages (S&W): payments made to employees of the institution for work performed.

scholarship: the process of advancing knowledge.

scientific method: the process by which scientists, collectively and over time, endeavor to construct an accurate (ie, reliable, consistent, and nonarbitrary) representation of the world.

scientific review group: a group of highly regarded experts in a given field convened by NIH to advise NIH on the scientific merit of applications for research grants and contracts. Scientific review groups are also required to review the ethical aspects of proposed involvement of human subjects. Various kinds of scientific review groups exist and are known by different names in different institutes of the NIH (eg, Study Sections, Initial Review Groups, Contract Review Committees, or Technical Evaluation Committees).

scope of work: the description of the work to be performed and completed on a research project.

senior personnel: professional personnel who are responsible for the scientific or technical direction of project.

single-masked design: typically, a study design in which the investigator, but not the subject, knows the identity of the treatment assignment. Occasionally, the subject but not the investigator knows the assignment. Sometimes called "single-blind design."

social experimentation: systematic manipulation of or experimentation in social or economic systems; used in planning public policy.

sponsor: the organization that funds a research project.

sponsor-investigator: an individual who both initiates and actually conducts, alone or with others, a clinical investigation. Corporations, agencies, or other institutions do not qualify as sponsor-investigators.

sports injury epidemiology: includes studies of injury patterns among athletes. These studies will generally encompass large-scale data collection and analysis. Surveys and questionnaires may be classified in this category but are more likely to come under the observation/informational studies category (see also *epidemiology*).

SRA: Society of Research Administrators.

statistical significance: a determination of the probability of obtaining the particular distribution of the data on the assumption that the null hypothesis is true. More simply put, the probability of coming to a false positive conclusion. If the probability is less than or equal to a predetermined value (eg, 0.05 or 0.01), then the null hypothesis is rejected at that significance level (0.05 or 0.01).

stipend: a payment made to an individual under a fellowship or training grant in accordance with pre-established levels to provide for the individual's living expenses during the period of training.

surveys: studies designed to obtain information from a large number of respondents through written questionnaires, telephone interviews, door-to-door canvassing, or similar procedures.

task order agreement (TOA): a legally binding document authorizing work and appropriating funds as a supplement to a basic contract.

teaming agreement: an agreement between two or more parties to participate in a research project or teaching activity.

technical data: recorded information, regardless of form or characteristic, of a scientific or technical nature. Often referred to as the "science" of a proposal.

tense: (grammatical) relates a verb's relation in time.

terms of award: all legal requirements imposed on an agreement by the sponsor, whether by statute, regulation(s), or terms in the award document. The terms of an agreement may include both standard and special provisions that are considered necessary to protect the sponsor's interests.

theory: a generalization or series of generalizations by which we attempt to explain some phenomena in a systematic manner.

therapeutic intent: The research physician's intent to provide some benefit to improving a subject's condition (eg, prolongation of life, shrinkage of tumor, or improved quality of life) even though cure or dramatic improvement cannot necessarily be effected. This term is sometimes associated with Phase 1 drug studies in which potentially toxic drugs are given to an individual with the hope of inducing some improvement in the patient's condition as well as assessing the safety and pharmacology of a drug.

therapy: treatment intended and expected to alleviate a disease or disorder.

total direct costs (TDC): the total of all direct costs of a project.

truth: the state of being the case, fact; or the body of real things, events, and facts; actuality.

unilateral award: an award made by a sponsor to an organization without considering competitive proposals. Unilateral awards are most often made when unsolicited proposals receive favorable treatment.

unsolicited proposal proposals: proposals submitted to a sponsor that are not in response to an RFP, RFA, or program announcement (see also *investigator-initiated proposal*).

variable (noun): an element or factor that the research is designed to study, either as an experimental intervention or a possible outcome (or factor affecting the outcome) of that intervention.

voice: (grammatical) action of a verb.

voluntary: free of coercion, duress, or undue inducement. Used in the research context to refer to a subject's decision to participate (or to continue to participate) in a research activity.

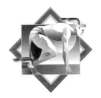

Index

BUILD *Your Library*

This book and many others on numerous different topics are available from SLACK Incorporated. For further information or a copy of our latest catalog, contact us at:

Professional Book Division
SLACK Incorporated
6900 Grove Road
Thorofare, NJ 08086 USA
Telephone: 1-856-848-1000
1-800-257-8290
Fax: 1-856-853-5991
E-mail: orders@slackinc.com
www.slackbooks.com

We accept most major credit cards and checks or money orders in US dollars drawn on a US bank. Most orders are shipped within 72 hours.

Contact us for information on recent releases, forthcoming titles, and bestsellers. If you have a comment about this title or see a need for a new book, direct your correspondence to the Editorial Director at the above address.

Thank you for your interest and we hope you found this work beneficial.

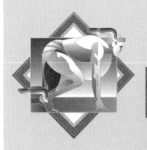

Expand Your Library
With These Exceptional Texts!

Other Exciting Books in the Athletic Training Library *Include:*

Title	Author	Book #	Price
❏ Professional Behaviors in Athletic Training	Hannam	44094	$24.00
❏ The Athletic Trainer's Guide to Strength and Endurance Training	Wiksten	44310	$24.00
❏ Current Topics in Musculoskeletal Approach: A Case Study Approach	DeCarlo	44345	$24.00
❏ Reimbursement for Athletic Trainers	Albohm	44086	$24.00

Subtotal $____

NJ and CA Sales Tax* $____

Handling Charge $ 4.50

Total $____

Name: _____

Address: _____

City: _____ State: _____ Zip Code: _____

Phone: _____ Fax: _____

Charge my: ❏ AMERICAN EXPRESS   ❏ MasterCard   ❏ VISA   Account#: _____

Exp. date: _____ Signature: _____

Prices are subject to change. Shipping charges may apply.
*Purchases in NJ and CA are subject to tax. Please add applicable state and local taxes.

CODE:4A687

Mail Order Form To: SLACK Incorporated
Professional Book Division
6900 Grove Road
Thorofare, NJ 08086-9864

Call: 800-257-8290 or 856-848-1000
Fax: 856-853-5991
Email: Orders@slackinc.com

Visit Our World Wide Web: www.slackbooks.com